"Fornay is a Master!"

Reviews

"He created the products, trained the experts, and traveled the country celebrating the beauty of black women. This is the book we've been waiting for. Fornay is a master."
—Susan L. Taylor, Editor-in-Chief, *Essence* Magazine, author of *In the Spirit* and *Lessons in Living*.

"Before black women knew which way to turn, where to look to affirm their beauty, and find the tools to enhance their beauty, there was Alfred, setting the pace.
—Constance White, Style Reporter, *The New York Times*; author of *Style Noir*

"Alfred Fornay has exemplified perfection in the beauty and fashion industry for 25 years. His style, élan and foresight have been emulated by countless others. Congratulations Fornay!"
—Naomi Sims, superstar model, Naomi Sims Cosmetics, author of *All About Health and Beauty for the Black Woman*.

"This book marks Mr. Fornay's leadership as the fashion and beauty authority for all African-American Women."
—John Ledes, Publisher, *Beauty Fashion Magazine*, and *Cosmetic World Newsletter*.

"Mr. Alfred Fornay's new book is a detailed, yet intimate skin care and make-up guide that every woman must have. An internationally-known beauty authority, Fornay blesses us, once again, with worldly beauty secrets that will help African-American women hit the new millennium beautifully and totally confident. Thank you, Mr. Fornay."
—Renee Minus White, Fashion & Beauty Editor, *N.Y. Amsterdam News* and President, *A Time to Style*.

"I have read the rest, now this book is the best. A realistic and entertaining approach to make-up and skin care. This book will be a valuable asset to every woman's reference library."
—Smiler Haynes, Senior Vice President, Barbizon, Boston, Massachusetts

"With this how-to guide, Alfred Fornay maintains his role as the beauty industry leader. He gives African-American women exactly what they need (from the inside out) to maintain a flawless complexion and enhance their natural beauty.
—Yvonne Rose, Senior Vice President, Edgar Morris Corrective Skin Care; author, *Is Modeling for You? The Handbook and Guide for the Young Aspiring Black Model*

Dedication

This book is dedicated to all women, past, present, and future,
who strive for excellence in their work, family,
and personal grooming. You have taught me to
respect and appreciate your ageless beauty.

Quote

Beauty is ageless, neither young nor old, but eternal.

t.r.

The African-American Woman's Guide to Successful Make-up and Skin Care

By former creative director for Revlon cosmetics
(Polished Amber Collections)
and marketing manager for Clairol
Alfred Fornay

First Edition

Amber Books
Los Angeles, CA   Phoenix, AZ

The African-American Woman's Guide to Successful Make-up and Skin Care

by Alfred Fornay

Published by:
Amber Books
1334 E. Chandler Boulevard, Suite 5-D67
Phoenix, AZ 85048
E-mail: Amberbk@aol.com

ALL RIGHTS RESERVED

© Copyright 1998 by Alfred Fornay

Library of Congress Cataloging-in-Publication Data

Fornay, Alfred.
    The African-American woman's guide to successful make-up and skin care /
    by Alfred Fornay.—1st ed.
    p.   cm.
    Index included
    ISBN 0-9655064-2-8
    1. Skin—Care and hygiene. 2. Cosmetics. 3. Beauty, Personality. 4. Afro-American women—
    Health and hygiene.   I. Title.
    RL87.F667   1998
    646.7'26'08996073—0021   98-21455
                                                                        CIP

10 9 8 7 6 5

First Printing January, 1999

Table of Contents

Acknowledgments

To my supportive sisters Beverly and Elizabeth, nieces, Sharmyn, Julie, Darla, Carla, Sherry, and nephew, Troy.

Mentors:

John H. Johnson
Benjamin Wright
Elsie Archer
Dr. Alfred Sloan
Hurley Phillips
Joseph Merriweather
Rose Morgan
John Ledes
Anthony B. Colletti

John Ledes, Joan Bowser, Bob Tate, Edward Lewis, Clarence Smith, Susan L. Taylor, Ionia Dunn-Lee, Marcia Ann Gillespie, Mike J. Bramwell, Byron Barnes, Constance White, Brian Basil Daley, Tony Rose, Naomi Sims, Alex, Valerie Bennett, Earle Holman, Ashley Hall, John Blassingame, Eddie and Grace Phipps, Edythe Karr, Sybil Gooden, Fred Dillon, Iman, Emmitt Dudley, Gwendolyn Nicholas, Carolyn Florence, Brian Hayes Copeland, Georginia G. Hill, Terry Ivory, Kelly Rollins, Bernice Coleman, Wanda J. Baskerville, Gloria Pflanz, Darrin Patrick, D'angelo Thompson, Lawrence Burchall, Kelvin Wall, Kendal Aegri, Sherry Bronfman, Audrey Bernard, Barbara Harris, Lee Willard-Stoffman, Evelyn Cunningham, Dr. Gloria Yoate, Bernice Calvin, Milton Scott, Wentworth Christopher, Bert Emanuel, Sheila Evers, Regina Fleming, Aunt Lois, Walter Greene, Therez Fleetwood, Ronald Lihurd, Alan Price, Roy Hastick, Yvonne Rose, Ruth Sanchez, Emel Lindsay Cross, Jessica Harris, Mary Garthe, Betty Johnson, Bernice Whistleton, Ernest Lee, Joan Murray, Tony, Michael, James Harris, Smiler Haynes, Rudy Townsel, Kathleen Myer Lane, Winston Isaacs, Jacqueline Champagnie, and Kowan Choi.

A special acknowledgment:

> Tony Rose, Publisher and Editor
> Terry Ivory, Editorial director
> Marie Dutton Brown, Literary agent
> Lisa Liddy, Cover and interior design
> Wayne Summerlin, Cover photo
> Alvaro, Illustrator
> Shonnette, Cover models make-up artist
> Yvonne Rose, Cover photo production coordinator
> Therez Fleetwood, Cover photo design
> Ashley Hall, Fashion stylist
> Jatawn Avanti, Cover models fashion stylist/dresser
> Roger Gary, Cover models designer
> Cover models: Cecily Witcher, Judith Riley,
> Ericka T. Moran, Greer Alexander
> Wayne Parham, Before and after photos
> Before and after models: Darlene Guinty and Everyday People
> Models' Troupe, Rabiya Dumas, Karima Henderson, Lena
> Nicholson, Cindy Gabbidon

As always, the **Publisher** gratefully acknowledges those whose time, patience, help, and advice have contributed to the success of our literary efforts:

> Erline Belton; Philip and Anjie Herbert; Felicia Rose and Kate Saylor; Florence Price; Regina Thomas; Elnora Marie Fleetwood-Miles; Yvonne Marie Fleetwood; Kevin Anthony Fleetwood, Jr.; Keva Victoria Miles; Angelita Miles; Aten-ra Prince Miles; Isis Elnora Jewel Miles; Kay Bourne; Cassandra Latney; Therese Fleetwood; Jamila White; Wayne Summerlin; Lisa Liddy; Rodney J. McKissic; Carol Herbert; Rachael Girard; Tom "Satch" Sanders; Darryl and Lorraine Sanders; Sharon Thompson; the IBBMEC; the Nation's African-American bookstores; our wholesalers and distributors; the black media; Yvonne Rose, whose love and friendship for the illustrious Alfred Fornay brought him to Amber Books; and Alfred Fornay who knows black women, and loves black women everywhere.

Foreword

Al Fornay's first work on beauty and grooming appeared in the *New York Times Magazine* in 1979, under the supervision of Patrica Petersen, then fashion editor. The article marked the first recognition of the huge African-American color cosmetics market.

Mr. Fornay emerged as one of the recognized authorities on fashion, beauty, and grooming. A graduate of the State University of New York's Fashion Institute of Technology and the City College of New York, with degrees in merchandising and marketing, Mr. Fornay has influenced the marketing and sales strategies of major cosmetics firms such as Fashion Fair, Clairol and Revlon. His training seminars for sales personnel and beauty consultants helped establish these companies as leaders in beauty and grooming for the African-American woman.

While traveling and presenting his seminars throughout the United States, as well as in Canada, London, Paris, and the Caribbean, Fornay developed the unique ability to anticipate the fashion and beauty needs of African-American women and men. He was among the first to perceive their desire for quality. Al Fornay helped his readers and advisees to feel and look better.

Fornay's coupling of language with graphic visual images soon had publishing houses seeking his flair for design and service marketing. Mr. Fornay helped the Johnson Publishing Company to establish their Fashion Fair Cosmetics line in Marshall Field's, Bloomingdale's, Carsons, Rich's, Robinsons, J.L. Hudson, Jordan Marsh, Nieman Marcus, Nordstroms, Macy's, and others. Mr. Fornay served as beauty editor at *Ebony* magazine, the first such post conceived to train black women and men in fashion and grooming techniques.

Fornay helped Johnson Publishing Company launch EM: *Ebony Man* magazine, and served as its editor-in-chief. He also served as the first male beauty editor of *Essence* magazine. And at McGraw-Hill, for *Business Week Careers* magazine, he was a contributing writer in fashion and beauty, an indication to young career seekers that dressing for success is a must.

This book marks Mr. Fornay's leadership as The Fashion Authority for all African-American women.

John Ledes, publisher,
Beauty Fashion magazine and *Cosmetic World* newsletter

Preface

After more than twenty-five years in the beauty business and having read hundreds of beauty books, I write this second book for women whose skin color ranges from the middle to the darker end of the spectrum because much of the information relating to these skin colors is confusing and often dead wrong.

Although I focus on African-American women, there are millions of other women whose coloring falls into this range: African, Caribbeans, Asian, Hispanic, and so on. If you are one of these women, this book is for you. It is about the health and beauty of your skin, its maintenance, its treatment, and its make-up. It is about the application of color to your skin and your nails. This is a "how-to" book for the person of color, whether she's manager of a small service store or an executive of a multimillion-dollar corporation. It is for the secretary of a five-person office and the editor of a major magazine. And perhaps most of all, it is for the housewife whose jobs are many and whose hours are ongoing. The book is for all women of color who want to look great and take better care of their skin.

Make-up and adornment, particularly the use of color, has a unique significance to black women. The use of make-up is a socioreligious, socioeconomic, and sociopsychological statement as much as it is a beauty choice. You will find some black women going to a cosmetic counter, looking at a photograph of Tyra Banks, Jada Pinkett, Iman, Toni Braxton, Halle Berry, Diahann Carroll, Angela Bassett, Vanessa Williams, and Whitney Houston and saying, "Oh, I would love to look like that."

A beauty advisor or cosmetologist then attempts to make the woman up to "look like that" and the woman looks at herself in the mirror, saying, "Oh no! That's not me." More than likely, the cosmetologist is stunned by this reaction and wonders—well, what does the woman really want?

The photograph does not reflect the reality of the woman at the counter. If she is a churchgoing woman, she probably only wears some foundation, shaded powder, tint-type lipstick, and little else. But if she is a top executive in the record industry, then she might be fully made up with color.

A woman's use of make-up relates to her sense of self and how she interacts with the world. Many African-American men don't like their wives using much make-up and color, and this, too, has an effect on how these women appear. In fact, more than 65 percent of the 16 million African-American women in the United States have never put color on their face. (A surprising statistic that should have cosmetics companies wetting their lips!) The question is, though, why don't they wear color and how can they be persuaded to? The make-up section of this book addresses this question and gives the black woman make-up color options that will comfortably suit her sense of self, style, and needs for home, church, social events, and work.

Many cosmetics companies—both black (special market companies) and white (general market)—have done outstanding research and development on how make-up relates to black skin. I will introduce you to their products and the research. Foremost among these companies is the black-owned Fashion Fair Cosmetics Company, but it is not alone. Naomi Sims, Black Opal, Iman, Interface, Sacha, and Patricia French of Gazelle Cosmetics and the Flori Roberts organization have done outstanding research, and they produce quality lines for black skin. In this book you will learn how to evaluate the quality of their lines and the many other beauty products filling the shelves of department stores and chain stores and pharmacies. You will discover how to choose what works best for you. You will learn how to address your own needs, not those of sales personnel, and be secure in your selection of color for your skin and nails. You will be able to determine your skin type and what colors are appropriate for each season. You will know what corrective beauty products to buy and what regular skin-care regimen to follow. By the time you finish reading this book, you will know the state of the art in the beauty industry and how to use that knowledge to your advantage.

I believe that every black woman is beautiful: She just needs to know how to present her beauty. After reading this book, you will be able to do just that. As Naomi Sims often says, "an ugly woman is a lazy woman."

You Are Born Beautiful…

African-American women are beautiful. Some women of color are born beautiful, but a much larger percentage have made themselves even more beautiful thanks to a skillful use of cosmetics.

For the past ten years, professional cosmetics educators have crisscrossed our nation teaching and instructing women of color in the proper application of cosmetics for their faces: Byron Barnes, Roxanna Floyd, Ellie Winslow, Reggie Wells, Sheila Evers, James Harris, Katara, Ricci, Bert Emmanuel, Lumus Hamilton, Lazarus, Ashly Hall, Kirk Norris Harris, D'angelo Thompson, Jonathon Romania and more recently Sam Fine and Christopher Michael.

We have all taught young and mature women that when properly applied, make-up can bring radiance to your complexion and smooth, conceal or camouflage your features. It can even change the shape of your face. All of the professional beauty educators advise this, but make-up must be used with wisdom and discretion. That little touch of color here and pat of powder there can be read like a billboard, telling the world about a woman's fashion savvy, her personal grooming habits, and her good taste.

Susan Taylor, Iman, Dee Simmons, Erline Belton, Yvonne Rose, and Therez Fleetwood, are six out of billions of women who are born beautiful, including you. They were selected for this book to represent women from all over the world. Their flawless skin and dedicated use of skin care products and make-up have only enhanced their natural beauty. Combined with intelligence, education, spirituality, and a professional image, these women are champions in every way.

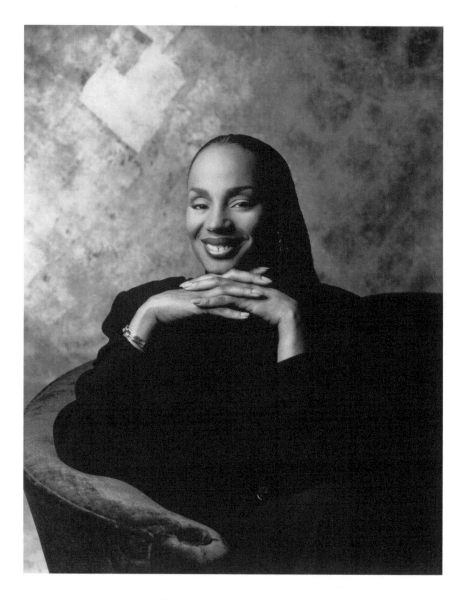

Susan L. Taylor

Senior Vice President & Editor-In-Chief, *Essence* Magazine

As a newly divorced, single mother, armed with only a high school diploma and cosmetologist's license, Susan L. Taylor joined the *Essence* fashion and beauty team in 1970 as a freelance beauty writer. One year later she was named Beauty Editor, and the following year her position was expanded to include fashion.

Since becoming Editor-in-Chief in 1981, Susan Taylor has guided *Essence* through a period of phenomenal growth. Her efforts have been rewarded with numerous awards and honors and a monthly readership of more than 7.5 million people.

Taylor was host and executive producer of *Essence,* the country's first nationally syndicated Black-oriented magazine show, which ran for four seasons in more than 60 U.S. markets as well as in several Caribbean and African countries. In that role she helped bring new and positive images of African-American men and women to the television audience. She was elected a Vice-President of Essence Communications, Inc., in March 1986. In June 1993 she was appointed Senior Vice-President. She is the executive producer of the annual Essence Awards and with a team oversees the Essence Music Festival, which takes place over the July 4th weekend in New Orleans and has been the largest gathering of Black musical talent in the world.

Her acclaimed monthly editorials, "In the Spirit," led her to the publication of her first book, *In The Spirit. The Inspirational Writings* of *Susan L. Taylor* in 1993. Her second book, *Lessons In Living* was published two years later; and her third book, *Confirmation: The Spiritual Wisdom That Has Shaped Our Lives,* co-authored by her husband, Khephra Burns, a writer and producer, was published in 1997.

Susan L. Taylor has become one of the most sought-after speakers in the country. Her personal commitment to help empower Black women and the poor has made her an avid supporter of a host of community-based organizations nationwide to which she donates her time to actively participate in fund-raising activities.

She's a member of the National Association of Black Journalists, the American Society of Magazine Editors and The Magazine Publishers Association. Her many honors include honorary doctorates from the nation's first Black college, Lincoln University, Delaware State University and Spelman College. She holds a B.S. in Sociology from Fordham University and is currently studying for her Masters in Divinity at Union Theological Seminary in upper Manhattan.

Her daughter, Shana, married former New York Knicks great Bernard King, and Susan is now the proud grandmother of Amina Suzanne.

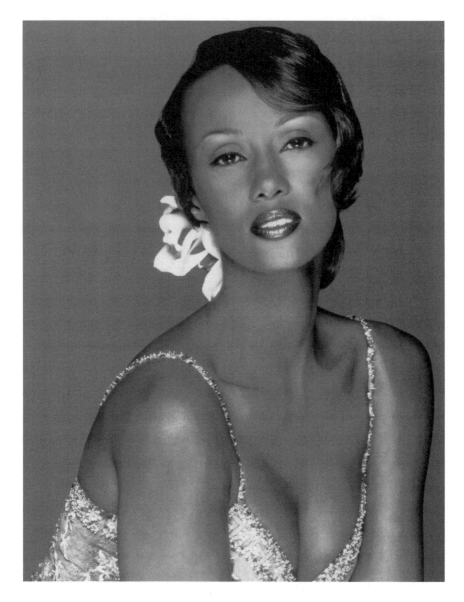

Iman

Profile of a Model/Actress in a New Role

Iman, an accomplished model and actress, who has graced the covers of magazines worldwide has been cast in a new role—the creative force behind her signature Cosmetics and Skincare Collection. *"Throughout my career, I had to learn to create make-up that looked good on me by being a good chemist,"* she explains *"I decided to introduce my own line because I realized that there wasn't a product on the market that met my needs or the needs of all women of color."*

Although the 43 year-old Somalian born beauty will continue to pursue her acting career—the Iman line is more than just a celebrity endorsement. She is involved in every aspect of the business—product development, package design, marketing, promotion and advertising. She has assembled a team of experts and advisors to ensure that her company utilizes the newest ingredients and advanced technology to develop superior products for women of color.

The IMAN introduction will also redefine current cosmetic marketing terminology. Until now, terms such as 'woman of color' and 'ethnic' have been associated with products developed for African American women. *"I believe that women of color, are the women of the world—Native American, Hispanic, Asian, Indian, African and Middle Eastern. These women live right here in this country,"* Iman points out, *"It's time to address the concerns of this invisible consumer because today's minorities are tomorrow's majority."*

Simply introducing a make-up line was not enough for Iman, she believes that skincare is equally important. *"Many women have become too dependent on color systems. If you can't walk out of the house without make-up and feel great about your skin, you have problems,"* she says. *"We have to start by dispelling the myths—we're not made of steel. Sunlight, pollution and stress affect our skin, too."*

In her new role, Iman is striving to create an environment where education and communication become the focus. *"I want the consumer to tell us what her needs are rather than us telling her what they ought to be,"* she points out. *"My main goal is to eliminate the constraints associated with beauty. I'm not telling anyone that I can make them look like a model, but I can make them look their best."*

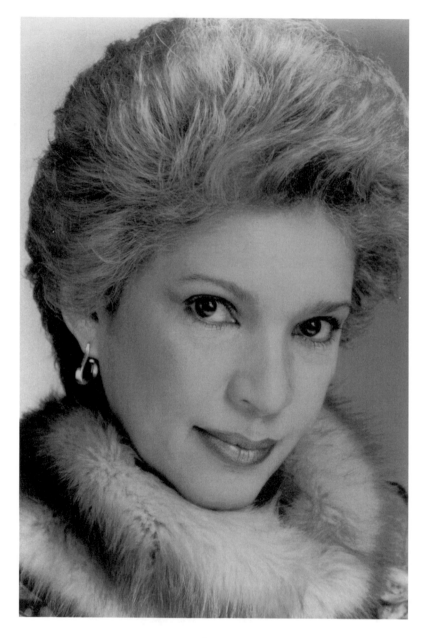

Dee Simmons

Vice President, Ophelia DeVore Associates and
Executive Director, Grace Del Marco Models

Business Executive; born in New York City, Dee attended Evander Childs High School, City College of New York majoring in Psychology and Business Administration and Manhattan Community College majoring in Entreprenuership. She then decided to make modeling her career.

Dee has been awarded Miss Sepia, and has won Miss Empire State, Miss Beaux Arts, and Model of the Year titles, to name a few. Dee was the first model of color to be a principal in a TV commercial in the United States for Artra Cosmetics. Early in her career Dee joined Ophelia DeVore Associates, Inc. as an instructor in the modeling school and as one of Grace Del Marco's top models.

Presently, Dee is Vice President of Ophelia DeVore Associates and the Executive Director of Grace Del Marco. In her role as director, she has been responsible for launching the careers of some of today's top Black models, while continuing to remain a top model herself. Dee is a world traveler; Producer of Fashion Shows and Model Competitions and sales promoter for Special Event Programs.

While directing Grace Del Marco is her primary concern, Dee occasionally steps back into her modeling role. She has been seen in TV Commercials for Oldsmobile, Chrysler Plymouth and the covers of Johnson Publications, *Sepia, American Salon, Black Hair Beauty & Lifestyle* and *Essence* magazines.

While she has been active in the fashion/modeling community, Dee is also very active in the civic community. She is a member of the National Association of Women in Media, a member of the Affairs Committee for the Freedom Fund Drive and with the NAACP. She has also received community service awards for her work in Anti-Narcotic Rehabilitation, and is the recipient of many Special Achievement Awards.

Throughout her career, Dee has been a positive image in the Black community. While her work with Grace Del Marco is quite demanding, she still finds the time to share her expertise by lecturing at schools and for organizations. Dee is currently the Producer & Host of her TV Cable Show "The Dee Simmons Show". She is a firm believer in commitment, a fact to which all of her students and models can attest to.

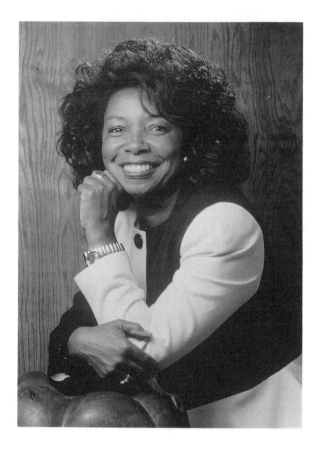

Erline Belton

President and Founder of The Lyceum Group

Erline Belton is the President and Founder of *The Lyceum Group,* a consulting firm whose major focus is to influence societal and workplace re-thinking which honors principles based in truth-telling. Her focus has been in the US and internationally. Her life work is to be of service to other's in their search to create effective results-based organizational legacies and to explore personal legacies with intention. Her most recent international assignments were in South Africa and Tanzania. She has been a senior executive for the past 18 years.

She has held multiple teaching appointments which included the University of Massachusetts, Tufts University, Wheelock College, and

Harvard University. She also worked for the Harvard Center for Social Policy and Change.

As a consultant, Ms. Belton's expertise in business and human resources gives her a unique combination of knowledge and skills for assignments focused on senior executive coaching, board development, human resource management and strategies, organizational assessment and realignment, and AIDS in the workplace strategies. Currently, her focus is on working with senior executives, leadership teams, and boards in private, public, and non-profit sectors. Her current interest is in the area of leadership and legacy creation and its relationship to building value-based systems in corporations, non-profits, and communities to ensure human well-being and justice to achieve economic growth.

Ms. Belton is active as a national and international speaker. Topics include creating leadership through legacy to build inclusive organizations, organizational transformation, diversity and human resource strategies, and AIDS in the workplace strategies, using truth-telling as the framework. Examples of previous speaking engagements are: UNESCO— Paris, France; Harvard Business School; The American Red Cross; First Chicago National Bank; Ford Motor Company Engineering Conference; US Department of Currency; Simmons Graduate School of Management; and The White House.

Presently, Ms. Belton serves on the Boards of Directors of the following non-profit organizations: Civil Rights Project Inc.; Women's Foodservice Forum; American Social Health Association; Wheelock College; Concord Center for American Studies; and the Boston Chapter of the American Red Cross.

Her corporate Board appointments include Unique Casual Restaurants, Inc., Personal Physician Care, Inc., and D'Ventures Inc.

Ms. Belton's formal education includes course study at Radcliffe and the International Executive Organization Development Program at Columbia University. She received her Bachelor of Arts and Masters in Education at Tufts University.

In January, 1990, Ms. Belton was featured in an *Ebony* magazine article entitled, "*100 of the Best and Brightest Black Women in Corporate America.*" She has been featured in *New Cleveland Woman* and in multiple human resource magazines. She was honored by the Museum of African American History of Boston, MA, in November, 1990, which included her portrait in an exhibit entitled, "Local Women Who Make A Difference in Boston."

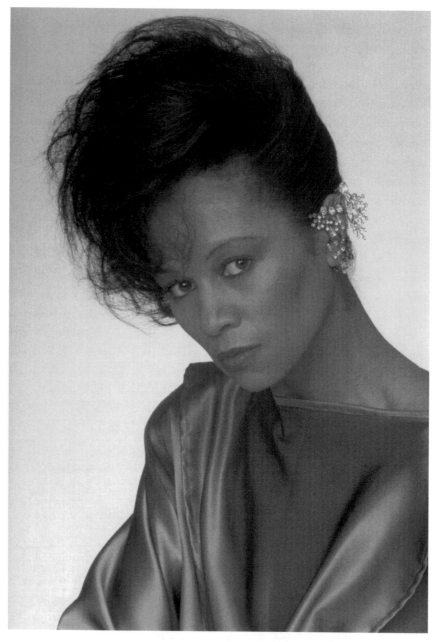

Yvonne Rose

Author of *Is Modeling for You?*
The Handbook and Guide for the Young Aspiring Black Model

Yvonne Rose, fashion model, journalist, and author of *Is Modeling for You? The Handbook and Guide for the Young Aspiring Black Model*, has spent most of her life in the fashion and beauty industry. She excelled as a beauty consultant and sales manager for Fashion Two Twenty/Lady Finelle Cosmetics, and later, as the Senior Vice President of Edgar Morris Skin Care, Inc. Having acquired a degree in Business Management, she opened an image consulting firm on Boston's prestigious Newbury Street. Soon after, Yvonne received her cosmetologist's license, and became a make-up artist for Fashion Fair Cosmetics and for (PBS) Public Broadcasting Television.

During that same time period, Yvonne joined the Grace Del Marco Agency and worked as a professional model with major fashion designers, taking her from her hometown of Boston to New York's 7th Avenue and to Europe. Her love of modeling expanded to teaching at such notable New York schools as Ophelia DeVore, Barbizon, and John Robert Powers. This led her into fashion commentary and fashion show production as the creator of Canadian Club's Black Designers' Showcase.

She has been Editor for Blac'tress/Black Hair Care, Fashion Editor for *CLASS* Magazine, and Contributing Editor for *Black Elegance* (BE), *Sophisticates Black Hair Care, Sisters in Style, Unique Hair and Beauty, Hype Hair* and *Right On!* magazines.

Since the release of her book, *Is Modeling for You?*, Yvonne has received numerous requests for guidance from aspiring models, teachers, and agents and has begun a "Modeling Consultant Service." As the "Models' Authority" she has coordinated and directed numerous self-help seminars for young people. In addition to her business ventures, Yvonne believes in giving back to the community and supports many local and national organizations.

She is the Youth Director and a member of the National Council of Negro Women (NCNW) and the NAACP. She is also a Board Member of Black Women's Task Force, the Co-director for the Hal Jackson's Talented Teens International Scholarship Competition, and a member of National Association for Female Executives (NAFE).

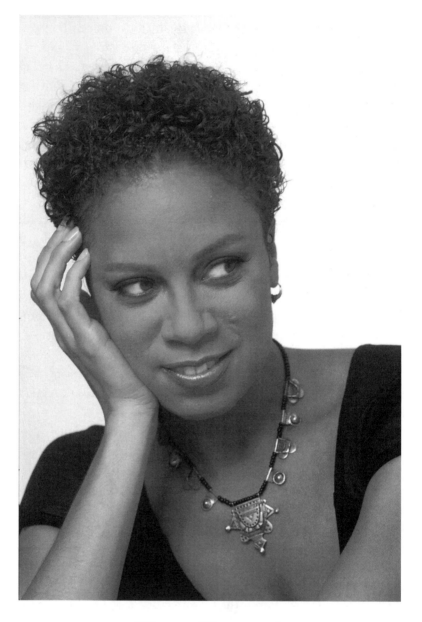

Therez Fleetwood

Fashion Designer

African-American brides have long sought to add cultural touches to their wedding attire. It was Therez Fleetwood's desire to fill this neglected market niche that prompted her to create the Therez Fleetwood Bridal Collection, a unique line of gowns which combine African fabrics and regional influences, with European cut and silhouettes. "African-American culture is a hybrid of both African and European traditions and styles," says Fleetwood, "but for a long time, we've had to choose between either traditional African or European attire for our wedding ensembles. My dresses bring together both of these cultures in a way that is very fashion-forward.

Fleetwood uses fabrics such as Nigerian Ashoke cloth (which has metallic threads woven in patterns similar to Kente cloth) and Guinea brocade to create her highly tailored gowns. The detailing in her designs is inspired by the dress of west, sub-Saharan, and northern African countries. Fleetwood also incorporates a mixture of fabrics with hand beading, or trim sewn onto the dress in detailed, Afrocentric designs. A trademark of her wedding gown is that each comes with a matching crown, which has a detachable veil.

Since launching her collection in 1993, Fleetwood has quickly become known as the leading designer of Afrocentric bridal wear. Her gowns have appeared in *Essence*, *Signature Bride*, and *Black Elegance* magazines. She designed the only wedding gown to be featured in the *Essence by Mail Catalogue* and she is one of 35 designers whose works were on display in the "New York Gets Married" exhibit at the Museum of the city in New York City.

Fleetwood, who attended the Fashion Institute of Technology (FIT) in New York, began her career in Afrocentric design in 1989 with the launching of her now defunct Phe-Zula collection. It was a well received line of casual, career, and formal wear, which was written up in an array of publications, including *Elle*, *Essence*, *Italian Glamour*, *Women's Wear Daily*, *The New York Times*, *New York Daily News*, and the *New York Post*. Under Phe-Zula, Fleetwood developed a long list of celebrity clientele, including Angela Bassett, Vanessa Williams, Queen Latifah, and En Vogue, whom she dressed for the 1991 Grammy Awards. That same year she took first prize at John Blassingame's fourth annual National Designer of the Year Awards. The popularity of Fleetwood's formal wear gained her a spot in FIT's tribute to the Black Fashion Museum in 1992 and her designs appeared in Fairchild Textbooks' *Survey of Historic Costume* in 1993. From 1991 through 1993, the designer's work was featured at the Detroit

Institute of Art's Bal African, the annual fund-raiser for its Museum of African art. Fleetwood has also created a line of clothing for Olmec Toys Imani fashion doll, and she designed the first Afrocentric costumes for Walt Disney World's Mickey and Minnie. As evidence of her success, Therez was awarded the 1995 Certificate of Achievement in graphic arts for creating children's educational cards. She was the main designer for the Avon Boutique, a quarterly catalogue which included home decorative, jewelry, and collectible items produced by Avon Products, Inc., targeting the African-American community.

In 1996, the popularity of her bridal collection caught the eye of executives at American Express and she was tapped to appear in the company's "Portraits" commercial, which featured five small businesses. Fleetwood's entrepreneurial spirit and the success of her designs earned her the Allstate Insurance company's 1997 "From Whence We Came: African-American Women of Triumph" award.

Fleetwood's gowns are made on request and her designs can be viewed by appointment. She can be contacted at (212) 714-8058.

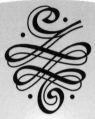

The African-American Woman's Guide to Successful Make-up and Skin Care

Chapter 1

How Your Skin Protects You

Your facial skin can be your best friend. It is your confidante. It is your protector. It takes all types of abuse, and yet it is quick and ready to forgive.

Your skin is a multifaceted creation that can't be duplicated by human beings. It keeps out the harsh external environment—that is, germs and bacteria—while it protects your vital organs. It helps maintain your body temperature by preventing heat from escaping too rapidly, which would lead to harm or even death.

Your skin is versatile and sensitive. It reacts to stress, pain, illness, pleasure, happiness, and to light and dark, hot and cold. It stretches and shrinks, wrinkles and unwrinkles. It needs minimal but regular, consistent, and thorough attention if you want it to show you at your very best. But for all your skin's strength and versatility, today it is under siege. It is bombarded by more natural and unnatural stresses than were ever intended.

Geography and the Seasons

Where you live has a direct effect on your skin, particularly on your face, for it is almost always exposed to the elements. Your face has an upper, or outer, layer of skin called the epidermis. This layer is what you touch and see when you look in the mirror. Actually, it is a series of layers, each somewhat different from the one above it but all with enough in common that together they make up the epidermis. Another name for this layer, owing to the shape of the cells making up the layers, is the "horny" layer (stratum corneum).

Although everyone has this outer skin layer, the thickness of the covering differs from person to person. African Americans have more layers to their epidermis than do whites. But even among blacks, the number of layers varies. Now you can understand why your face, to some degree, reacts differently to the forces assaulting it than do the faces of other women you know.

The outermost portion of the epidermis consists of dead cells. That is why sometimes, after washing your face and drying it with a towel, you may notice flaking skin on your forehead. Your face casts off this outermost layer of skin in pieces. As the outer layer is dispelled, an under layer takes its place. This is a constantly renewing process. Each outermost layer falls away when it has absorbed all the stress it can manage, and then the under layer takes its place.

While this surface action is taking place, the under layer is protected, waiting to supply your face with a new fighting army of cells. Beneath the epidermis is the germinating layer, but before discussing this lower layer, let's see what geography and climate can do to the outer layer of your skin.

If you live in a year-round warm region like California, then your skin will be affected differently than if you live on the East Coast, in a climate that has four varying seasons. Obviously, there is a difference in the amount of the sun and ultraviolet rays that will attack your skin, based on where your home is. But this is only the beginning.

If you live in a very sunny climate, then generally the office buildings are air conditioned year-round. The same is true when you fly in a pressurized aircraft. Whether it's in the sky or on the ground, air-conditioning draws humidity from the air and moisture from the skin. So, by the time you go from your dry office into a sun-drenched day, to bombard your skin with ultraviolet rays and further draw off moisture, your skin has really taken a beating. The skin is left dry, peeling, and if the exposure was too intense, with its under layers damaged.

The effect of just these two factors—sun and air-conditioning—is significant and potentially serious. This is the damage that sunburns do: you peel or you're left with leathery-looking skin. Worse, this constant negative stress breaks down the face's connective tissue, resulting in wrinkles and "aging." With steady damage, those wrinkles and lines around the eyes and mouth begin getting deeper and more prominent.

If you live in a seasonal climate, you might feel safer—and to some degree, that is true. But in the East, often there are major industrial complexes nearby that spew pollutants into the air. And wherever you live or work, your skin is exposed to automobile emissions and wind. Wind alone can strike at your skin and cause damage, but when that wind carries pollutants, the problem is intensified. The pollutants that cause acid rain destroy forests and crops, so you can imagine the struggle your outer skin layer has to protect your body.

Central heating, as well as air-conditioning, dries out the skin. This instrument of comfort adds stress to your face and brings on a premature aging process. To some degree, the effects of the seasons—even geography —may not be as dangerous to your face as is the modern technology we've created to make our lives more comfortable.

Other natural assaults come from germs, bacteria, and environmental impurities. These elements also must be prevented from getting below the skin's surface. So no matter where you live, your face contends with major stresses. More often than not, the outer layer stands up to these assaults—but at a cost: dryness, wrinkles and lines, and skin disorders. Your skin can't fight the "good fight" alone; it needs your help.

❦ Misinformation

Perhaps even more disturbing than the elements our skin is exposed to is the degree to which people are misinformed. Black and dark-skinned women and men have often been led to believe that their skin is built for the sun. Their African background is used as the factor to make this belief seem true. In fact, it is not true.

If you take a careful look at "blacks" living in the desert, or in comparably dry, hot regions like the Sudan, you will note that their bodies almost always are totally covered and very little of their skin is exposed to the sun. In contrast, people living in hot, humid areas are less apt to wear clothes—and rightfully so. Generally, the hot, humid areas have little if any direct pollutants, and the humidity in the air reduces the degree to which skin moisture evaporates. People who live in very humid climates don't peel; the skin of blacks and whites often has fewer wrinkles and they have faces that belie their age. The outer layer of their skin is moist and pliable, rather than dry and lined.

I've talked with women from Gabon and the Central African Republic, and they complain about how dry their skin becomes when they visit America. Their complaints have validity, since the humidity here is relatively low. A change in climate like this is often noticed within a few days or less. So remember—whatever your color, protect your skin or you will pay for the neglect.

Black skin has special qualities. As I noted earlier, it has more epidermal layers than white skin. To some degree, this means greater protection from the sun and those additional layers, black skin often appears and feels smoother. Black skin has more melanin (the dark pigment in the epidermis), which reflects more of the sun's rays, giving greater protection and reducing the drying process. But for all these positive qualities, black skin needs as much care as any other if it is to maintain its health and good looks.

❧ Devices of Protection

As previously stated, there are two upper layers to the skin: the epidermis and the germination layer, which together make up the skin's essential defense system. The outer layer has two essential ingredients helping it to do its job and maintain its "looks": water and sebaceous oils. These two elements—no matter how often you may have heard that oil and water don't mix—work together beautifully to support and protect the skin.

The epidermis needs water to keep it pliable, plump, and elastic. The body supplies that water through the cells. Later I will discuss diet, but for now I mention only that you need to drink plenty of water to maintain healthy skin. The sebaceous glands produce oils that travel upward and cover the surface of the skin. The oils act as a defensive shield and a reflector, holding the skin's surface moisture in and also keeping the skin soft, pliable, and unbroken. However, once moisture is drawn from the outer layer, the oils cannot help restore the skin's youthful quality. Only water will do the job. If you soak a piece of dry skin in oil, for example, it

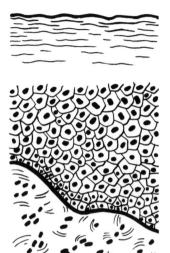

The upper layer of epithelial tissue, the under layer of germinating tissue, and the dermis, with regular blood cells.

will not soften. It will not soften even if you use sebaceous oil. The oil is not the softener, water is. Remember this principle when we focus on products for your skin-care regimen.

The Germinating Layer

Beneath the epidermis is the germinating layer. Actually, this is the deepest layer of the epidermis, resting on the corium, which is also called the derma, or true skin. But the germinating layer is so different from the rest of the epidermis, and should be nurtured so differently, that I present it as though it were a distinct layer. It consists of a single row of columnar cells, in which young cells develop and move upward to the surface.

The top cells making up the germinating layer move upward while others remain, protecting the corium beneath. The germinating layer does not maintain itself on water or oils, but is nourished by the blood circulated to the skin. This layer of cells is nourished as are cells in the rest of your body, through proper nutrients. This is why what you eat and don't eat, what you take into your system and what you don't take into it, will

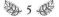

Epithelial tissue, the dermis, and a pore opening with a sebaceous gland extending upward to the skin's surface.

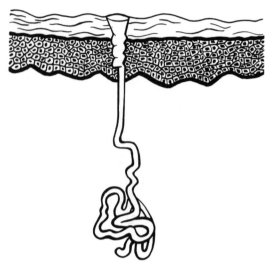

show in your face. What gets into your circulatory system will be seen, one way or another. Drinking alcohol will show, smoking will show, drugs will show, birth-control pills will show. A healthful or poor diet will show. Your skin is an indicator of your state of health. Moreover, your state of health will either help or prevent your skin from doing its job.

❦ The pH Defense

Those sebaceous glands have another defensive purpose besides holding in the skin's moisture. They maintain what is called an acid mantle across the skin's surface. Healthy skin is slightly acidic. It is believed that skin with a tendency toward alkalinity (the opposite of acidity) is more likely to become infected and have skin disorders. The pH factor of healthy skin (a tendency towards acidity) works as a defense, warding off infection and disorders that affect the skin's ability to both do its job and save the body from having to fight beneath the surface as well. So when you see products proclaiming to return the skin's pH factor, don't automatically accept or reject them, but know that the pH measure is important.

I have deliberately not discussed the skin's corium, or derma, since commercial products cannot affect it. Your genes, diet, and cosmetic surgery are its primary influences. So you can readily understand that the epidermis and germination layers with the sebaceous glands are the skin's primary, effective defense against the environment, both human—and nature-made. The "fall off" defensive process of the outermost layer of the epidermis serves two vital functions: (1) the older and drier cells are removed, and as the layer of the cells falls off, (2) the environmental impurities, bacteria, and pollutants on or in them are removed.

This self-renewing process is ongoing, with little visible evidence when your skin is young and healthy. However, when your skin in neither young nor healthy, then the process works less effectively, with the noticeable results of lines, wrinkles, cracks, and peeling. But with help and knowledge, you can retard the aging process and keep your skin healthy and youthful-looking.

❧ Water—A Key To Youthful-Looking Skin

Even though the outer layer of the skin receives a continuous supply of water from the inner layer, the amount provided is limited at any given time. Thus, the outer layer is often short of water when it may need it most. For example, if the skin's loss of water to the atmosphere exceeds its upward supply, then the skin is in danger of going dry. If you don't use a sunscreen or moisturizing guard, the extreme dry conditions in such areas as Arizona, New Mexico, and the desert in California can have a dangerous effect on your skin.

❧ The Aging Process

If you look at the skin of an older person, particularly if it has been neglected or abused, you will find evidence of structural change. The dead, outer layer of the epidermis is thicker and therefore drier. In part, this is because the epidermis begins to produce a slightly different type of cell.

Furthermore, these cells stick together with greater adhesion and are not shed as readily. The outer layers of dead skin begin to build up thicker and thicker atop the lower, living layers. These outer layers have not only less water or moisture in them but also less capacity to hold water. Unless their moisture capacity is increased, the outer, now thicker layer becomes dry and wrinkled. This causes creepy lines to appear, with the ends of the cells curling up, leading to roughness.

During this aging process, the oil glands decrease in function, with the decline greater in women than in men. Also, the surface guard of oil, whose function is to hold moisture in the skin, does not work as well. Without its water retention, the skin loses its pliability and softness. Finally, the outer layer may hold up to the point where rough, red spots appear and discolorations show up on black skin.

Suntanning and the Aging Process

Tanning is a device the skin uses to protect its delicate inner layers. This increase in pigment, brought about through exposure to sunlight, by and large is temporary; the suntan disappears in time. However, during the aging process, there is a tendency for these pigments to increase, causing the skin to become darker and, in some instances, blotchy. These darker areas usually appear on the hands and face. Often they are called age spots or liver spots, and they are permanent. Actually, these are the result of suntanning combined with the aging process. People who stay out of the sun have fewer, if any, liver spots.

Lines, Wrinkles, and Spots

If you were able to take a look at the skin's lower layer—the dermis —you would notice elastic fibers. The dermis cannot regenerate itself as can the epidermis, or outer layer. Any damage done to the dermis results in degeneration and the formation of scar tissue. This means there is a structural change, no matter how slight. It is this under layer that is reasonable for the resiliency of your facial skin, whether smooth and unlined or rough and wrinkled. The dermas is composed of layers of living tissue, and this tissue is permeated with elastic fibers—reinforcement rods that help keep the skin taut. If damage is done to these rods, sagging and wrinkles are often a result.

With the aging process, the under layer has a tendency to degenerate, often causing these fibers to break into many pieces. Their supportive effectiveness is then gone, and the dermis is incapable of "standing up" by itself. In some places, the structure caves in and the outer surface falls into the crevices. These are the face's grooves, lines, and wrinkles. The skin around the eyes and on the neck is the most likely to show these aging signs first, with the rest of the face showing the effects later.

The blood vessels, which are also in the dermis, expand with age and even may break, causing little capillary discolorations.

❧ Protect Those Layers and Look Youthful

Remember: it is what happens in the dermis that most often creates the sense of facial aging. When damage occurs in the dermis, and happens throughout the facial area, the effects are permanent. Only cosmetic surgery can rebuild or stretch the perception of new life and youth. No matter how much care is given to the face, some structural changes will occur. But these changes can be kept to a minimum with proper care and preventive treatment. This means that paying attention to both the outer and inner layers of the skin is essential.

❧ Nutrition and Your Skin

Let's look at the things you can do to achieve more healthy, youthful skin. For instance, there are healthful enhancement amino acids such as cysteine; vitamins A, B, B-complex, and PABA; and the minerals zinc and selenium, which , combined in the right dosage, can help retard the aging process.

The following vitamin therapy is recommended by Dr. Mitchell Kurk, a family practitioner in Lawrence, New York. Dr. Kurk treats skin conditions nutritionally as well as with medication, and he believes that drugs should only be a last resort. This is his formula for the healthy adult over thirty years of age. Remember: always check with your physician before taking any vitamin regimen beyond an approved over-the-counter supplement.

VITAMIN	QUANTITY
Vitamin A (60% beta-carotene)	25,000 I.U.
Vitamin C	1,200 mg
Vitamin D3	100 I.U.
Vitamin E	400 I.U.
Thiamin	100 mg
Riboflavin	50 mg
Niacin Niacinamide	190 mg
Vitamin B6	100 mg
Polate	800 mcg
Vitamin B12	100 mcg
Biotin	300 mcg
Pantothenic acid	500 mg
Iodine	200 mcg
Magnesium	500 mg
Zinc	25 mg
Selenium	200 mcg
Manganese	20 mg
Chromium	200 mcg
Molybdenum	100 mcg
Potassium	99 mg
Calcium	500 mg

Dr. Kurk recommends this formula as a supplement to a healthy diet, and says that it is excellent for more than just your skin. However, I repeat: no diet or health program should begin without a thorough medical checkup first by a licensed physician. Dr. Kurt's formula meets the minimum needs indicated by the latest research, as appropriate for enhancing your health and retarding the aging process.

Dosage direction: 2 tablets, 3 times a day (6 tablets a day).

Cost: $30.00 for tablets, $5.00 for shipping and handling; $35.00 total order.

For more information, you may contact: Dr. Mitchell Kurt, 310 Broadway, Lawrence, New York 11559, 516-239-5540.

Some "Don'ts" and "Do's"

Now let me give you some "don'ts" and "do's" for healthier black skin. (I place the "don'ts" first here because they can undo all of the "do's.") Remember: the effects of these bad habits are more noticeable on black skin than on white, whereas the good habits are helpful to everyone.

☞ Don'ts

☐ 1. *Don't smoke.* Smoking cuts down on the amount of oxygen getting to the tissues, resulting in impaired circulation and a breakdown or pre-aging of skin tissue. The results are dry lips, lines and wrinkles, dull ashy complexion, and sagging skin. Nicotine is a toxic substance—a poison.

☐ 2. *Don't consume excessive amounts of caffeine.* Usually you think in terms of coffee and tea; however, sodas are the greater culprit. Caffeine increases stress, which can show on the face.

☐ 3. *Don't sunburn.* Ultraviolet rays from the sun dry out the skin. The deeper the tan, the deeper the moisture loss. Dry skin loses its flexibility, softness, and suppleness, giving a dry pre-aged look. Without sufficient moisture—even creams can only do so much good—the skin will line and wrinkle. It may take years to see the damage, but once done it is just about irreversible.

☐ 4. *Don't drink alcohol.* Those who consistently drink too much decrease their food intake, resulting in improper nutrition, including a lack of vitamins and minerals—especially B1, which is necessary for healthy skin.

☐ 5. *Don't take too many or long baths in the winter.* Long baths in the winter remove the protective oils from the skin, which are helping to keep the necessary skin moisture in the cells for suppleness. Once the oils are removed, moisture is drawn off. Even oil baths are not as effective as your natural oils, but do use them after a bath.

☐ 6. *Don't use petroleum jelly and its by-products, cocoa butter, or oil as a facial skin moisturizer.* Oils are not moisturizers, and will not make your skin soft and supple. They will hold existing moisture in, but unfortunately the oils, if heavy or thick, can clog the pores, causing eruptions. Oils will definitely cause a shine, often giving a false impression of oily skin when in fact the skin may be dry. This is particularly true for those who are swarthy or dark-complexioned.

❑ 7. *Don't leave make-up on overnight.* Make-up left on too long can irritate skin, clog pores, cause eruptions, etc.

❑ 8. *Don't stay in overheated rooms unless absolutely necessary.* Over heated rooms usually are dry and will draw the moisture from your skin, helping dry it out.

❑ 9. *Don't overeat.* Being overweight is unhealthy and affects the condition of your skin. The stored fat accumulates peroxides, which are immune-system depressants, leaving the body more open to attack, including allergies. An unhealthy body affects the long-range quality of your skin, particularly the dermis.

☞ Do's

❑ 1. *Do exercise.* Proper exercise causes perspiration and the cleansing of pores, removing impurities from your system. It also increases blood flow to the surface, bringing needed nutrients. Ten minutes of peak exercise a day can be healthy and effective.

❑ 2. *Do drink six to eight glasses of water daily.* Your system needs water; your cells need water to replace lost water and maintain skin moisture.

❑ 3. *Do use a water filter.* You should drink nonchlorinated, nonmetalionized water. These are oxygenates, which bring on preaging symptoms. Use a filter that draws off these minerals and trace elements from your water. Filters are cheaper in the long run than bottled water and give water that is equally palatable. Your cooking and ice-cube water should be as pure as your drinking water.

❏ 4. *Do have a full-length mirror in your bedroom.* Make sure you face the mirror nude, from all angles. This helps keep you on your diet as you see the positive changes and helps get you on a diet if you don't like the additional poundage.

❏ 5. *Do use nutrient supplements if you drink alcohol.* I mentioned the loss of vitamin B1 and poor diet that usually accompany much drinking. This admonition is not to suggest approval of drinking but to reflect an awareness that many may not stop and yet will want some type of protection. See the section that follows for recommendations.

❏ 6. *Do eat properly.* Supplement your meals with the nutritional vitamins, minerals, and amino acids. Certainly, a vegetarian diet with nutrition supplements is healthful and produces healthy skin, but as a general rule, eat raw and steamed vegetables, fish, and chicken. Limit your intake of red meat; candy, desserts, and sugar in general; tea and coffee; and sodas. Take cod liver oil, zinc, vitamins C and E, and lecithin.

❏ 7. *Do weigh yourself regularly.* Every week, get on the same scale in the same room at the same time.

A Nutritional Supplement for Drinkers

The following nutritional supplement is recommended for moderate drinkers. It was prepared by Durk Pearson and Sandy Shawn, authors of *Life Extension.** They list the total dose per day, to be divided into three doses and taken with meals:

SUPPLEMENT	QUANTITY
Vitamin A	1,200 I.U.
Vitamin B	.12 g
Vitamin B2	24 mg
Vitamin B3 (niacin)	72 mg
Vitamin B5	24 mg
Vitamin B6	60 mg
Vitamin B12	60 mcg

Vitamin C	.36 g (at least three times as much vitamin C as cysteine)
Vitamin E	120 I.U.
Choline	.36 g
Cysteine (not crystal)	.24 g
Zinc (chelated)	60 mg
Selenium	30 mcg

Consult your physician before starting such a program, and do not follow this formula if you are diabetic, suffer from ulcers, or drink heavily.

*Dosage extrapolated from data in Life Extension a *Personal Scientific Approach: Adding Years to Your Life and Life to Your Years* by Durk Pearson and Sandy Shaw, copyright©1982. Reprinted by permission of Warner Books, New York.

Chapter 2

How To Touch Your Face

Have you ever thought about how you touch or should touch your face? If you are like most women, you probably have not. I consider how to touch your skin so important that I make this a first "how to" section in this book. You can use all the correct products and colors, and follow the best nutrition, but still damage your face because you touch it improperly. By "touching your face," I refer to how you attend to it with your hands, such as when you clean it, apply toner, or blend on astringent, moisturizer, and other like products.

Clean Hands, Directed Movements

You should try to touch your face only when your hands are clean. Your facial skin has enough to deal with without your accidentally adding dirt and bacteria from your hands. There is a proper technique for touching your face, based on how the muscles and skin on your face are attached and how they work.

You should always use your fingers in the direction that reduces stress—that worked with, rather than against, your facial muscles and skin. The following illustration shows the direction your fingers should move on various parts of your neck and face. When cleaning or massaging your neck, move upward with your hands or fingers to the chin line. When

15

touching your face, use your fingertips in a circular motion, moving outward from the nose to the hairline except around the eyes.

Remember, although you have five fingers, they are not equally appropriate for your face. The ring finger is most serviceable. It is your weakest finger; yes, it is even weaker than your little finger. Test it and you will see. You want to use a light touch, so use the ring finger, partially when working in the eye areas, which have the thinnest layers of epidermal skin. (That is why age lines show themselves faster and more often in these areas.)

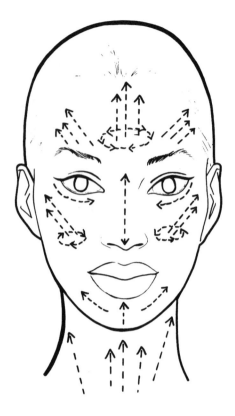

The Eye Area

When cleansing or massaging your face around the eyes, always work from the outer temple inward toward the bridge of the nose. You should move in this direction because the facial muscles around the eyes are suspended from the temple toward the nose. Going in the opposite direction stretches the skin and muscles, and risks damage. Once damaged, there is little that can be done, other than to have injections of collagen or silicone to fill the damaged area. Most dermatologists, though, are reluctant to have black women take these injections because black skin is easily bruised and retains dark spots, either or both of which could result from such injection. I repeat: always use the ring finger under your eyes.

The Rest of the Face

Use the fingertips of your first three fingers for your cheeks, and for your forehead, move in a circular motion out to the hairline. The chin is massaged with the first three fingers of each hand, moving from the center of the chin outward with a gentle, rotating motion.

❧ Gently Stimulate As You Touch

Whenever you touch your skin, you should try to gently massage it at the same time. The stimulation from gently slapping and massaging the face is very helpful. This form of touching causes the blood to rush upward to the surface, replenishing the skin while drawing away impurities and leaving a nice glow. Another positive is that this action reduces facial stress as well as stress throughout your body. Relaxing the facial muscles may reduce those lines in the forehead and around the mouth or prevent them from getting deeper.

If you have oily skin, however, you should stimulate your skin less often than if you have dry, because frequent massaging will bring additional oil to the surface.

❧ Your Make-up Tools

Now that you know how to touch your face, whether you are massaging or cleansing it, you need to learn which cosmetic instruments to use when applying make-up to your face.

There are approximately seven tools that most women may use, and we will look at them one at a time: Face cloths, buff puffs, loofahs (sponges), facial tissues, cosmetic cotton balls, cosmetic swabs, and facial brushes.

Facecloths

Most people, including women, use a facecloth to wash their face and body. Unfortunately, many women do not think about the abrasive quality of their facecloth. Many cloths, after being wet from use, will dry and harden overnight, with the cloth's nap turned into a myriad of hard little bristles. When you use this cloth to scrub your face, the results —whether initially visible or not—are that you bruise and often cut the outer layer of skin, particularly around the eyes. So while cleansing you have abused your skin when your intent was just the opposite.

The guiding principal here is to show loving care to your face. Be gentle and kind. Buy and use only pure cotton facecloths because they dry softer and maintain a soft nap.

When you use a cotton facecloth, wrap it around your hand or fingers like a mitten. Work your finger, covered by the cloth, over your face as described earlier. Don't rub hard to stimulate or remove flaky skin. If you want to stimulate your face, use the massaging and slapping technique described. It will not bruise, irritate, or damage your skin or the capillaries below the surface. Don't forget: work the eye area gently, and move the cloth from the temple to the bridge of the nose. Do the forehead with a circular motion, moving outward and upward to the hairline.

Buff Puffs

Buff puffs are made of synthetic materials. They are used in washing, scrubbing, and stimulating the face. I have a general aversion to the buff puff because black women have to be so careful in using them. All too often, because of their harsh synthetic quality, the buff puff cuts or causes abrasions to the skin, resulting in a burn that may darken and become a spot. If you use a buff puff to stimulate, you must be extraordinarily careful and use it in the most gentle fashion.

If you use a buff puff, do it no more than once or twice a week, and them only with kindness and gentleness. Buff puffs should never be used by black women with acne.

Loofahs

Loofahs, or luffas, are natural sponges, but they are harder and have a look of straw until they are soaked in water. There are other natural sponges, such as silk sea sponges, which are very soft and generally are used for applying make-up. When choosing a loofah, buy the softest and least abrasive one you can find. There is no doubt that, after use, your face will have a radiant glow and the look of good health, but this could be deceiving. It is possible the abrasive quality of even a soft loofah may irritate the skin in the process of stimulating the blood flow. It is best suited for using on your skin from the neck down.

Before using, always thoroughly soak the loofah in water, so it is as soft as possible. If necessary, err on the side of caution. When your face is at risk, don't use a loofah regularly; reserve it for these special occasions, and then use it gently.

Facial Tissues

There are two major "don'ts" when you think of using paper tissues on your face. The first is that you don't use tissues that contain wood pulp. Tissues applied to the face should be soft. Generally, the more expensive tissues are free of wood pulp, which, when it touches your face, can cut, scratch, or split the delicate skin mantle without your feeling or immediately knowing it. This damage can result in bruising or darkening of the healed scratch, and can even develop into a keloid (thickening of scar tissue).

The second caution is that you don't use tissues if you have excessive facial hair, skin eruptions, and so on. The fibers of the tissue may cling or get into skin openings, causing infections, discomfort, and additional problems. What is most interesting is that these concerns probably seem unnecessary because you may think they haven't happened to you. Unfortunately, the damage generally is not visible, unless you really look for it. The situation is the same as when you smoke: the injury to your body is not seen initially but by the time it is, the damage has been done.

As I consistently plead, err on the side of caution. You have everything to gain and nothing to lose. When working with tissues, use them gently and use only those free of wood fiber, when your face is smooth and free of pimples, bumps, and other blemishes.

Cotton Balls

When using cotton balls, think of them as if they were tissues. The same potential problems from using paper tissue exist for cotton balls. Buy only the pure natural-fiber cosmetic cotton balls or pads. Avoid synthetic cosmetic "cotton" balls. How can they be man-made and still be cotton? They cannot. They are damaging to your skin, so be careful; check them out.

Real cotton balls are excellent because they are sanitary. You use one, throw it away, and get another. Cotton balls are particularly good when applying toners, astringents, and fresheners, or in cleansing the delicate tissue around the eye.

Cosmetic Swabs

Your swabs should be of the best brands and of pure cotton, spun properly so that the fine cotton hairs are intact and flat on the head of the swab. This is important because loose fine cotton hairs can damage the skin, particularly when the swabs are used to clean the corners of the eyes. Properly designed pure-cotton swabs, either round or flat, are excellent for applying eye shadow, color application, and for cleansing around the nose and under the eyes. Again, as you use them in these areas, make sure that you work from the temple inward toward the bridge of the nose.

I must mention here that swabs should be used in the outer ear and not placed in the ear channel. I know this point does not relate to your face, but always when I am interviewed or on tour, women mention using swabs for their ears as well as their face. There are better ways to clean your ear channel than to place a swab in it.

Facial Brushes

I like most of the brushes on the market today, and I consider them equal in value to pure-cotton facecloths for facial use. I am particularly fond of brushes made of gentle natural or man-made fibers. Some are sponge types while others are very soft bristle form. The one type I recommend black women avoid is the rubber facial brush. Black skin bruises and marks easily, and a rubber facial brush may cause a friction burn, resulting in a bruise and discoloration.

❧ The Best Tool For Each Job

For all of the tools mentioned, the materials you should always feel safe using on your face are your own clean fingers. You can control them better than any of these other cosmetic tools. Next best are the natural cotton facecloths and facial brush, excluding the rubber bristled ones. Don't forget: when using a facecloth, wrap it around your fingers so that you are using your fingers as though they were inside a cotton mitten. When using a facial brush, be gentle and use the same motion you would if you were using only your fingers.

Tissues, cotton balls, and swabs should all be made of pure cotton. Swabs and balls are for limited service: swabs for under eyes and in crevices around the nose; cotton balls for applying toners, astringents, and fresheners, and for cleansing. Tissues have the most limited use, mainly for cleaning or toning the face. Yet all these cosmetic tools can be serviceable if they are of fine quality and are used with care.

☞ Don't Forget

☐ 1. Use the fingers, and particularly the ring finger, when cleansing or touching the face.

☐ 2. The ring finger should be used in the eye area, and the movement should be from the temple toward the bridge of the nose.

☐ 3. Finger motion should be circular and outward to the hairline except for under the eyes.

☐ 4. Fingers on the neck should move upward to the chin line.

☐ 5. When stimulating the face, use the fingertips with a gentle slapping or patting motion in the directions outlined.

☐ 6. Wrap your pure-cotton facecloth around your fingers and touch your face for cleansing as though your fingers were in a cotton mitten.

☐ 7. The same movements you employ in using a facecloth should be used when working with a facial brush (not rubber).

Chapter 3

Your Skin Type and How to Care For It

Up to this point, I have worked with you on how to touch your face and what materials to use when cleansing, toning, and stimulating your face. You may be thinking, "That's fine, but what do I cleanse or wash my face with? Soap, creams, cleansing lotions?"

Before I can help you choose the right products to put on your face, you need to determine your skin type. You have to organize what you know about your face in order to become an effective cosmetic consumer, in terms of both value for your money and what is correct for your skin. Remember: what you put on your face *can* hurt you.

This chapter has three parts. The first helps you determine your skin type. The second discusses appropriate products for your skin type. The third applies the information conveyed in Chapter 2 to help you use the right products on your face. When you finish this chapter, you will know all the basics for using the methods described throughout the book.

Determining Your Skin Type

A black woman can have more than one skin type. For instance, you may have a basic skin type that is altered by outside factors. Many women find that there are seasonal or other reasons for their skin type to change. Their skin may become dryer or oilier, or may be more sensitive than usual, based on whether it is spring/summer or fall/winter. Some women find that they have skin changes based on their menstrual period or as a result of dieting, alcohol consumption, birth-control pills, and even smoking. Additionally, drug abuse, allergies, and aging can affect your skin condition.

These effects are particularly noticeable on black skin because black skin is deceptive—beautifully so—but deceptive. The amount of melanin and carotene in black skin will often cause light to reflect off, or appear to, rather than to be absorbed, as it is on much lighter or on white skin. If there is any perspiration on the nose or chin, the center of a black face may appear shiny. This shiny quality gives the impression that the skin is oily, when actually it may not be. In fact, the skin could be dry.

A Few Simple Rules

You can look at your skin and recognize what type it is if you know how to look. Make sure you have sufficient light, meaning that it approximates daylight, and be sure the light covers your entire face. No part of your face should be in shadows. First, you will notice your T-zone. This area comprising your forehead down the bridge of your nose, and from your nose to your chin.

If you are light or dark-skinned, you may notice light reflecting off the T-zone as you look in the mirror. Look to the left and then to the right of the T-zone, and compare how your skin looks. See if there is a different amount of light reflected on the left and right sides of the T-zone, compared to the T-zone itself.

If the sides of your face and the T-zone are the same, with clean hands touch first your forehead, then the tip of your nose and your chin. If there's perspiration, wipe it away. At this point, there is more testing to do, but you probably have normal skin. If you feel oil, touch the sides of your face; if they also feel oily, then your skin is oily.

When you look at your face, note any areas that appear different, either patchy, rough, or discolored. Patchiness and roughness are often signs of dry skin; however, your face could have areas that are dry and others that are normal or oily. And this situation can change with the seasons, your health, and possible pregnancy.

Clear Your Mind and Clear Your Face

This technique for determining your skin type may seem complex, but I want you to rid yourself of all those old and untrue beliefs you may have had about your skin type. I want you to realize that skin classification requires close attention to your face as well as other conditions affecting your body. I want you to forget the notion that all you have to do is look to the T-zone or type your skin once, and the job is done forever.

For example, so many women buy the wrong products for their faces, thinking that they have sensitive skin because their faces break out. This is money wasted and keeps a skin problem unresolved.

Check Your Skin Type Twice a Year

Evaluate your skin type twice a year: once during spring/summer and once during fall/winter. But don't do it at the very beginning or end of the season. Do it a few weeks into each time, and use common sense. If the change in season is very abrupt, evaluate your face sooner; if the change is almost imperceptible do it a little later. When you change your clothes for the season, that is when to make your test. Of course, I don't mean when you change clothes to be color fashionable. I mean when you change for body comfort.

❦ The Skin-Typing Questionnaire

Here is the easy part that helps take the guesswork and confusion out of typing your skin. I have developed ten questions, the answers to which will help you determine what kind of skin you have. The chart on pages 26-27 shows these questions, with characteristics listed for four skin types: oily, combination, dry, and sensitive. Your answers to these ten questions can be matched to the corresponding characteristics. In some instances, there is only one description; in others, two or more situations characterize that skin type.

Remember, I have deliberately given up to four possible skin types. This is to force you to think in terms of that which is most usual, most noticeable. Certainly, we could refine the table further, but it would be valueless.

Questions to Determine

QUESTION	OILY
☐ 1. Before and after cleansing, can you see oil?	Always
☐ 2. Does your skin feel greasy or slick?	T-zone All over
☐ 3. If you bathe with deodorant soap, how does your face and body skin feel after an hour, without any type of moisturizer?	Oily foreheads, eyelids, nose, and chin
☐ 4. What do your pores look like?	Wide, enlarged all over
☐ 5. Do you have blackheads or whiteheads?	Many Summer problems
☐ 6. Do you break out?	Frequently
☐ 7. Do you peel or crack around the forehead, eyes, nose, mouth, lips, and chin?	No Summer Occasionally in winter, especially around nose and mouth
☐ 8. Does your skin look tight, smooth, and ashen?	Rarely
☐ 9. Does your cleanser and moisturizer sit on top of your skin or disappear immediately into it?	Never disappears
☐ 10. How do you react to sun?	Rarely burn, good tan

Your Skin Type

COMBINATION	DRY	SENSITIVE
Sometimes: Oily in spring/summer Dry in fall/winter	Rarely	Sometimes: Summer problems
T-zone	T-zone Summer	T-zone Sometimes
Slightly dry-looking in appearance and feel Jawline and around eyes in fall/winter	Taut, tight, and dry in feeling and appearance with ashen dull cast	Tight and shiny T-zone after first half-hour Sometimes in winter
Enlarged in T-zone, especially on nose, cheek, and chin	Almost invisible, fine pores	Noticeable in T-zone, fine elsewhere
T-zone problems Cheeks	Few Summer problems	Occasionally
Occasionally	Rarely Few in summer	Always Rashes and patches
Occasionally	Frequently Around eyes, forehead, mouth, lips, and chin, especially in winter	Occasionally Around eyes and nose
Sometimes Winter	Frequently, on forehead, cheeks, jawline, and chin	Rarely
Sometimes disappears	Always disappears immediately	Sometimes disappears
Slow burn, especially in summer	Burn easily without moisture protection	Burn easily without moisture protection

❧ Analyzing Your Skin Type

We classify your skin to help you buy products that are designed for your basic skin type. These products cannot be tailored to your exact skin, however. It is like fashion designing. If you have a personal fashion designer, he or she can tailor a pattern, and change it as your body changes, to produce clothes exactly for your body. However, when you go to the department store, no matter how upscale it is, you must choose an item from "the rack." It must be altered to fit you, and those altered measurements are made only in a few places. In cosmetics, there are no after-purchase refinements or tailoring. You take the product from "the rack" and use it as recommended by the beauty adviser, based on the skin-type information you have provided.

In recent times, the cosmetics and beauty industry has done an excellent and thoughtful job of researching skin types. The products they offer cover a wide enough range both to properly address your skin's needs and to enhance it while maintaining its health. You can analyze your skin type closely enough to achieve proper product selection. By reviewing the skin-type analysis chart on pages 29-30 you can use your answers to the skin-typing questions to determine your actual skin type. Based on which column most of your answers fall into, you will know your basic skin type.

❧ Your Skin-Care Regimen

Now that you have determined your skin type, you can think in terms of proper facial care. When I mention "facial care," be aware that you can only address the epidermis. There are no products that penetrate deeper. Remember: proper external care and proper nutrition are two keys to healthy, beautiful skin. If you add the third key—stress reduction—you not only will have healthy, beautiful skin but it will have fewer lines and your life expectancy will be extended.

Start now with a proper skin-care program. There are three basic steps to any quality skin regimen: cleanse, tone, moisturize. These are followed by a maintenance step, a special beauty procedure.

Skin Type Analysis

Question	Answer	Question	Answer
Oily		Combination	
I	Always	I	Sometimes: Oily in spring/summer Dry in fall/winter
2	T-zone All over	3	Slightly dry-looking in appearance and feel Jawline and around eyes in fall/winter
3	Oily forehead, eyelids, nose, and chin	4	Enlarged in T-zone, especially on nose, cheek, and chin
6	Frequently	5	T-zone problems Cheeks
		8	Sometimes Winter

Skin Type Analysis

Question	Answer	Question	Answer
Dry		Sensitive	
3	Taut, tight, and dry in feeling and appearance with ashen dull cast	3	Tight and shiny T-zone after first half-hour Sometimes in winter
4	Almost invisible, fine pores	4	Noticeable in T-zone, fine elsewhere
5	Few Summer problems	5	Always Rashes and patches
7	Frequently Around eyes, forehead, mouth, lips, and chin, especially in winter	7	Occasionally Around eyes and nose
8	Frequently on forehead, cheeks, jawline, and chin	10	Burn easily without moisture protection
9	Always disappears immediately		
10	Burn easily without moisture protection		

Cleanse

Select a cleanser that meets the needs of your type skin, then relax your face, massaging it as described in Chapter 2. See the following illustration. The cleanser will help remove the outer cells layer and the impurities imbedded in your pores. (Clogged pores are a major reason for skin eruptions or blackheads.) The cleanser should clean deep but gently.

When choosing a cleanser for use during the summer, women with oily and combination skin should think in terms of lightweight or light-textured products such as water-soluble lotions and gels. These clean gently and have less detergent, and less of a drying effect on the skin. In the winter, women with dry skin might look to creams and rich emollients.

Try more than one of these products for your skin type, because each will be a little different. When you find the cleanser you like best, stay with it until you type your skin again, when there might be a need for a change, or if your skin reacts to the product. Remember, though that when your skin reacts, it may not be to the cleanser. First look to your diet, drinking habits, menstrual period, oral contraception, or possible pregnancy. If these are all eliminated as the cause, look to stress. When it, too, is determined not to be the cause, look at the products you are using. But generally, if properly chosen, your cleanser will not be the cause. Of all products, skin cleansers are the most researched and tested.

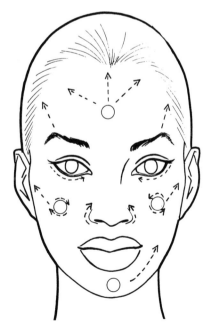

Step 1.

Cleanse, following illustrated direction of application.

Tone

Products used for toning the skin, which you may have heard of or have even used yourself, are astringents, skin fresheners, refining lotions, and clarifying lotions. A toner rinses off any cleanser or soap film on the face. But in our regimen it does even more than that. Its other purpose is to prepare your skin to receive a moisturizer. And it has yet another purpose. Do you remember that in Chapter 1 I mentioned the pH factor and the belief that the skin's natural acidity helps protect it from bacterial infection? A toner restores the pH to a proper level and corrects the balance of oil and water on the skin's surface.

A toner is particularly important for those women with oily, dry, or sensitive skin, for it will attend to their skin's balance needs. Look at the Beauty Resource Guide in the appendix and choose a toner suited to your skin type. Then apply it as shown in the following illustration.

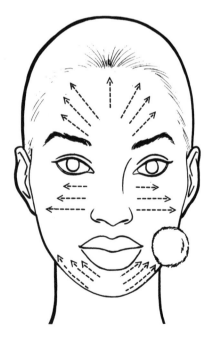

Step 2.

Apply toner, following illustrated direction of application.

Moisturize

Moisturizers do different things for different skin types. However, they will do the following for all skin types: become a sealer to hold skin moisture in (emollients) and draw moisture from the air to the skin to help keep it lubricated (humectant). If your skin is dry, then your moisturizer will lubricate and protect your face with an oil based mixture which adds necessary oil. If your skin is oily, then your moisturizer will be oil-free, for your skin has all the oil it needs. The moisture will also be water-based, fragrance-free, and dermatologically tested since such skin has a tendency to be sensitive. Apply the moisturizer as shown in the following illustration.

A moisturizer is a liquid or cream with two critical ingredients: a humectant and emollients. A humectant attracts and absorbs moisture in and on the surface of the skin as long as possible. They are either oil or non-oil substances in accordance with whether you have dry skin (oil-based) or oily skin (non-oil-based).

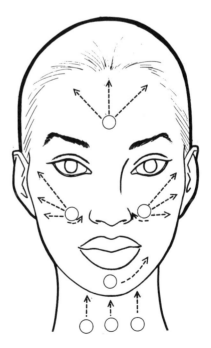

Step 3.

Apply moisturizer with fingers or applicator in the direction illustrated.

If you have combination skin, consider the time of the year and the condition of your body. If it's winter and your skin is dry in places (for example, on your jaw or chin), use a moisturizer for dry skin in those areas and one for normal skin elsewhere. If it's summer and your T-zone is oily, concentrate on a moisturizer for oily skin.

All too often, women who have dry skin apply mineral oil, petroleum jelly, or cocoa butter to the eye area. This suffocates the tissue around the eyes; it cannot breathe, and it swells and gets puffy. This is exactly what you don't want. Always use a specially formulated eye oil—a lightweight, refined oil cream for this delicate area. Massage the cream in, gently patting it on with your ring finger and working from the temple down to the nose. For oily-skinned women, I recommend oil-free eye preparations to lubricate this area.

A Special Beauty Step

The special beauty step is a maintenance one. Once or twice a week, based on your skin type, you should use an exfoliating lotion, cream, or gel. These exfoliates are for deep cleansing. They reach deeper into the epidermis than can your daily cleanser.

During general cleansing each day and evening, often specific types of problem skin—for example, very dry or very oily skin—require a super cleansing. Based on the season of year and your skin type, I suggest that you indulge in weekly deep cleansing and treatment. By "deep cleansing" I mean to cleanse, tone, exfoliate or mask, and so on.

If, for example, you have dry skin and it is wintertime, use a mask in spots, so as to deal exclusively with the problem area and leave the rest of your face alone. If you have oily skin and it is summertime, use an exfoliate and/or a deep-pore cleansing mask to rid your skin of dead cells and to unclog your pores.

When choosing a cleanser, make sure the ingredients are not harmful or abrasive to the skin. Some general cleaners contain grains which act as a mild exfoliate and skin stimulator. Often, the grains remove the outer layer of skin. But when the grains are chips of shells or nuts, they often have pointed, sharp edges that can scrape, split, and damage the outer layer of facial skin. Natural grains, unlike shells and nuts, are rounded and will not cut or cause such damage; they dissolve as you gently massage and scrub.

You may be thinking about one consideration I haven't yet mentioned: the eye area. This is the most delicate area, with the thinnest and fewest layers of skin. When cleansing, use the mildest nonabrasive cleansers and remember to use your fingers gently in this area and to move them from the temple toward the bridge of your nose.

Now that we have outlined the general skin-care regimen, let's get specific in terms of coupling your skin type with your specific skin-care regimen.

☙ The Oily Skin Classification

If your skin is normal to oily, there is a basic regimen to help you balance and control the oil. It's important that you drink eight glasses of water a day to flush your system of internal impurities and excess oil. Your oily skin systematically produces too much oil, day and night. If the surface sebum (sebaceous oil) is not removed at least twice a day, your skin mantle collects oil, perspiration, bacteria, and impurities that will cause problems—for example, clogged pores, blackheads, and acne.

Usually, oily skin is noticeably uneven in skin tone, light in the center of the face (T-zone), and slightly dark at the temples, outer cheeks, lower jawline, and chin. It is plagued with constant flare-ups and breakouts. Oily skin has visibly wide pores and a greasy, slick feeling. It can even appear dull.

A clean face is your goal. Oily skin must be washed at least once during the day and again before retiring. (The desired cleansing is at least three times a day, reapplying fresh make-up when convenient.) Your oily skin is not a problem when you know what to do. But you must plan your time and take care to meet your skin's requirements.

Day Care

PRODUCTS TO USE

PRODUCT DIRECTIONS

Step 1. Cleanse
Use lotion and liquid soap detergents formulated for oily skin. Nondeodorant soap bar (facial soap) also is recommended for oily skin. Use oil-free water-based products researched for black women.

Use tepid (lukewarm) water to rinse your skin. *I do not recommend a cream cleanser on oily skin during the spring/ summer months in any region.* Water-based cleansing lotions are fine if without mineral oil. (Lotion cleansers are excellent for removing stale make-up prior to deep-pore cleansing.)

Note: Acne oily skin is a medical problem and requires the attention of a dermatologist. Ask your dermatologist about products before you purchase. Gentle facial brushes are excellent but scrubs are best to help clean clogged pores. A natural fiber puff and non rubber cleansing brushes are recommended.

Step 2. Tone
Use a fragrance-free astringent and formula for oily skin. Skin fresheners and clarifying lotions formulated for oily skin are excellent for fall/winter.

Use lavishly; apply with cotton ball or pad and wipe until clean. Avoid the eye area. Also, don't use an astringent that has resorcinol, a skin-darkening agent.

Step 3. Moisturize
Use water-based, oil- and fragrance-free formulas for oily skin only.

Light moisturizers are water-holding agents that protect, retain moisture, and shield against the environment. Place 4 dots of moisture lotion at the forehead, cheeks, and chin and massage into skin.

No residue or tacky feeling should exist.

PRODUCTS TO USE	PRODUCT DIRECTIONS
For lips, a mineral-oil lip moisturizer is excellent. No oil-producing glands exist on top or bottom lips, so mineral oil can seal in and protect dry tissue against the environment. Oily skin types can have dry lips during all seasons.	Apply a cocoa butter, camphor, beeswax, lanolin, or petrolatum lip moisturizer directly from the tube or pat on your lips. This formula is for lips only, and is not appropriate for the facial area ever!

Evening Care

PRODUCT TO USE	PRODUCT DIRECTIONS
Step 1. Cleanse Step 2. Tone Step 3. Moisturize	Same as for day care
Special Night Care: Use a waster-based oil- and fragrance-free eye make-up remover.	Use product with a cotton ball or cotton eye pad to remove eye make-up. Rinse with tepid water to remove all traces.
Eye Treatment: Use formula for oily skin.	Sweep in gently with your ring finger from the outer corner of each eye toward the bridge of the nose.
Neck treatment: Cleanse, tone, moisturize, and apply night cream or anti-aging preparation.	Massage the formula into skin at the neck and throat area. See face chart, Chapter 2.

Weekly Care

PRODUCT TO USE	PRODUCT DIRECTIONS
Use a deep-pore exfoliate or scrub formulated for oily skin. Clay mask with conditioning properties is best for oily skin, especially in spring and summer, if fragrance-free.	Deep-pore cleansing dislodges imbedded dirt in the pores and removes the outer layer of skin-dulling dead cells. Cleansing grains are great, but avoid formulas with sharp particles, since they scratch and scar delicate skin tissue.

Your goal is oil control. You don't want to deplete the skin's natural oil, but you do want to kill the shine. Actually, there is an advantage to oily skin: African-American women with oily skin age less and at a slower rate, owing to the oily deposits deep in the layers of the dermis.

Here are some do's and don'ts for women with oily skin:

☞ Do's

❑ 1. Do drink eight glasses of water daily.

❑ 2. Do use only water-based, oil-free, fragrance-free products.

❑ 3. Do use astringents as often as you can—day and night as well as weekly.

❑ 4. Do use a clay mask at least twice weekly, spring/summer, and once a week in fall/winter.

❑ 5. Do avoid fatty foods.

👉 Don'ts

☐ 1. Don't use oil-based creams, lotions, or soaps.

☐ 2. Don't use acne-medicated cleansing pads as an astringent. You'll dry out areas around the eyes, temples, nose, and chin.

☐ 3. Don't use abrasive cleansing pads, buff puffs, or loofahs on your face frequently.

☐ 4. Don't use PURE alcohol, witch hazel, hydrogen peroxide, or concentrated lemon juice as an astringent.

❧ The Dry Skin Classification

If your skin is normal to dry, there is a basic regimen to help you maintain a balance between moisture and oil. It's important that you drink six to eight glasses of water a day to restore the body's moisture and to flush your system of impurities. You should also know that dry skin requires serious attention.

Coating and pore-sealing oils—such as baby oil, mineral oil, and petroleum products—do not condition or relieve rough, patchy, flaking, and sometimes uncomfortably itchy skin. The ashen skin will disappear when these coating and sealing oils are applied, but they clog the pores and allow particles from the environment to stick to the skin.

Dry skin can look dull and gray or ashen, be sensitive, and often be painful. Its fine pores can clog and break out. The problem areas are the forehead, lower cheeks, jawline, and chin. A dry, peeling nose can have fine dirt imbedded as blackheads and whiteheads on the side and tip, invisible and unnoticeable but sensitive to the touch. Dry skin reacts to extreme cold and hot temperatures, and suffers from a lack of both internal and surface moisture (dehydration) as well as from inadequate production of surface oil (sebum). Dry skin ages faster than oily or combination skin. The result can be premature wrinkles and crepey-looking lines around the eyes and mouth.

Day Care

PRODUCT TO USE	PRODUCT DIRECTIONS
Step 1. Cleanse Select a dry-skin oil cleanser if your skin is extremely dry, a rich creamy formula if your skin is moderately dry, and, if you are a soap-and-water person, a nondeodorant formula with rich emollients and conditioners designed for dry skin.	Tissue or rinse off. Massage gently, always moving upward and outward; see face chart in Chapter 2. Rinse with tepid water until your face is absolutely clean.
Step 2. Tone Use a non-alcohol toner for extremely dry skin or a low-alcohol toner for moderately dry skin.	Apply with a cotton ball or pad and wipe until all traces of surface impurities are gone.
Step 3. Moisturize Select a rich dry-skin emollient with moisturizers and conditioners specifically for dry skin. I prefer the fragrance-free tested formulas.	Smooth in gently from the base of your neck, massaging from the throat area upward to the hairline.
Your lips suffer in the winter. Use a mineral-oil lip preparation to trap and seal moisture on your lips. Medicated formulas relieve cracked, peeling, bleeding, and splitting.	Gently smooth in the penetrating emollient. Do not apply this formula to your face.

Evening Care

PRODUCT TO USE	PRODUCT DIRECTIONS
Step 1. Cleanse Step 2. Tone Step 3. Moisturize	Same as for day care.
Special Night Care: Use a no-tear, fragrance-free, dermatologically tested make-up remover.	Use product with a cotton ball or cotton pad to remove eye make-up. Rinse with tepid water to remove all traces.
Eye Treatment: use a rich light-textured emollient.	Sweep in gently with your ring finger from the outer corner of each eye toward the bridge of the nose.
Anti-aging treatment: use a night cream or anti-aging cell-renewal formula for your extremely dry, line- and wrinkle- prone skin. Mature dry skin may require a special firming cream or lotion to help soften and smooth the skin and restore a healthy glow.	Massage formula into skin on neck, throat, face, ears, and at hairline.

Weekly Care

PRODUCT TO USE	PRODUCT DIRECTIONS
Use a moisturizing cream to slough and peel off dry skin. (If you have thick facial hair, the peel-off type is not recommended.) Avoid clay or drawing formulas because they remove too much natural oil and moisture.	Apply a thin film of moisturizer over extremely dry skin before applying a gel peel-off mask. Cream the mask with healing conditioners—e.g., Aloe Vera.

Your goal is to replenish and maintain the balance of water and oil on your delicate skin surface. You want to rid the skin of dulling dead facial cells and impurities.

You must take every preventive step to lubricate and hold moisture on your skin. Harsh winter and summer air robs your skin of its natural moisture and oil. You can retard the deepening and lining of your face with proper care and with moisture-conditioning formulas that penetrate the layers of the epidermis.

Here are some do's and don'ts for women with dry skin:

☞ Do's

❏ 1. Do drink eight glasses of water daily.

❏ 2. Do use only oil-based, moisture-conditioning, dermatologically tested products.

❏ 3. Do use a cream mask for very dry skin.

❏ 4. Do ventilate your daytime and evening rooms. Humidifiers are an excellent way to control moisture.

❏ 5. Do use spot facial masks during summer and winter, applying them to problem areas only.

☞ Don'ts

❏ 1. Don't use astringents formulated for oily and combination skin.

❏ 2. Don't use abrasive, exfoliating granular-based masks.

❏ 3. Don't use deodorant-type soaps on your face. From the neck down, deodorant soaps are fine.

❏ 4. Don't use petroleum jelly, cocoa butter, mineral oil, or baby oil as a facial moisturizer, especially if you are going to wear a cream or liquid-cream make-up foundation. Cocoa butter and petroleum by-products are excellent for the lower body parts, however.

❧ The Combination Skin Classification

Your skin may be oily, dry, or sensitive in different areas, and it requires special attention in both summer and winter. There is a basic regimen you should follow to maintain a balance between moisture and oil. It's important that you drink eight glasses of water a day to flush your system of internal impurities and to restore the balance of water and oil on the surface of the skin.

When in balance, a combination skin can actually be normal. But seasonal conditions can affect combination skin to the point where it may be normal during one season and dry or oily during another. Additionally, stress, a dramatic weight loss or gain, dietary food changes, an irregular menstrual cycle, and aging can disturb the natural balance of acidity, moisture, oil, and dryness.

Skin eruptions, breakouts and patchy rashes can sometimes occur on your forehead, cheeks, and chin. Your pores are fine around the hairline, temples, chin, and jawline but visible in the T-zone. Your skin can be part oily and part dry at the same time, so you must select appropriate treatment products for areas of your face and time of year.

Day Care

PRODUCT TO USE	PRODUCT DIRECTIONS
Step I. Cleanse Use a liquid soap with mild detergent and facial shampoo properties. There are water-based lotions and nondrying facial cleansing soap bars designed for normal to combination skin.	Splash on water and rinse thoroughly with tepid water. Use the face chart in Chapter 2 for proper movement directions as you massage.
Step 2. Tone Use an astringent for oily zones in summer. Use a skin freshener for normal to dry zones in winter.	Dampen a cotton ball or pad and wipe until ball or pad is absolutely clean.

PRODUCT TO USE	PRODUCT DIRECTIONS
Step 3. Moisturize Use a lotion or lightweight soufflé-type moisturizer.	For summer oiliness, apply oil-free moisturizer all over, from neck to forehead. For winter dryness, apply soufflé-type moisturizer cream. Apply moisturizer with fingers or applicator in the direction illustrated on page 33.
For lips in winter use a moisturizer on both lips.	Apply directly from tube or pat on.

Evening Care

PRODUCT TO USE	PRODUCT DIRECTIONS
Step 1. Cleanse Step 2. Tone Step 3. Moisturize	Same as for day care.
Special Night Care: Use eye make-up remover for combination-type skin.	Use product with a cotton ball or cotton pad to remove eye make-up. Rinse with tepid water to remove all traces.
Eye treatment: use formulas appropriate for dry and oily eye zones.	Using the ring finger, gently apply eye preparation over and under the eye.

Weekly Care

PRODUCT TO USE	PRODUCT DIRECTIONS
Anti-aging treatment: use cell-renewal firming lotions or creams and night creams designed for dry and oily skin.	A few drops of this firming formula is applied to the problem aging areas.
Problem areas: use a clay mask for oily areas. A creamy mask with soft grains helps draw out toxins, heals, and firms and alleviates whiteheads and blackheads.	Spot-mask the oily areas twice a month in the summer and once a month in the winter for 6-10 minutes. Avoid applying clay mask to dry areas of the face.

Your goals are to treat, care for, and maintain your normal to combination skin. Summer emphasis is on the oily zones and winter efforts are on healing and conditioning the dry areas. Weekly deep-pore cleansing is important.

Here are some do's and don'ts for women with combination skin:

☞ Do's

❑ 1. Do drink eight glasses of water daily.

❑ 2. Do use oil-free products that are light in texture for the summer season.

❑ 3. Do choose skin fresheners and toners formulated for normal and combination skin, based on the season.

❑ 4. Do use products formulated and tested for normal and combination-type skin.

☞ Don'ts

❑ 1. Don't use the same product year-round. Your skin type changes dramatically. Observe your skin and note the oily and dry areas.

❑ 2. Don't use abrasive cosmetic tools over the entire face, especially in the winter months.

❦ The Sensitive Skin Classification

If your skin is sensitive, there is a basic regimen that will calm, balance, and alleviate discomfort. It's important that you drink eight glasses of water daily to rid your body of external impurities. Use fragrance- and oil-free products. Hypoallergenic or dermatologically tested products are applicable.

Your skin type has less tolerance of chemical substances and reacts to bad dietary habits, stress, hormonal changes, allergies, trauma, and impurities in the environment. It tends to be more dry in certain areas and may have frequent skin eruptions. Your skin may bruise easily and dark spots may be the result. Cosmetics companies have made excellent efforts to meet your sensitive skin-care needs, with products that are dermatologically tested to heal, soothe, and relieve your skin conditions and to improve your skin texture.

I recommend that you consult a dermatologist for treating extreme or severe sensitive skin conditions. And have a cosmetologist or beauty advisor do a patch test before you purchase a new product; you might even take a sample of that product to your dermatologist.

Day Care

PRODUCT TO USE	PRODUCT DIRECTIONS
Step I. Cleanse In summer, use a lotion, liquid soap, or facial soap bar. In winter, use a liquid cream or cream formula that is fragrance- and oil-free. Use products tested for black sensitive skin.	Massage liquid facial shampoo and lotion gently with your fingertips, using the face chart in Chapter 2. Rinse thoroughly. Tissue off or rinse off water-soluble creams.

PRODUCT TO USE

PRODUCT DIRECTIONS

Note: Do not squeeze acne pimples, or dark scarring may occur. Do not use harsh cleansers or scrubs. Do not aggravate overactive oil glands or eruptions. Preparations are on the market to correct young people's and adult acne. See a dermatologist.

Step 2. Tone
Use a skin freshener designed for black sensitive skin, with low or no alcohol or resorcinol. Skin fresheners fight bacteria, balance the oil and moisture levels on your skin, and refine the pores.

Wipe the entire face, avoiding eye zones, until a cotton pad or ball is absolutely clean.

Step 3. Moisturize
Use fragrance-free and oil-free treated lotions, or light, creamy soufflé-type moisturizers, that are formulated for black sensitive skin after liquid facial soap shampoos and toners. Fragrance- and oil-free moisturizers are water-holding agents to protect, condition, and smooth surface tissue.

In summer your skin does not need a coating or sealing of moisturizer. In winter apply a light film of cream.

Evening Care

PRODUCT TO USE	PRODUCT DIRECTIONS
Step 1. Cleanse Step 2. Tone Step 3. Moisture	Same as for day care.
Special Night Care: Use a no-tear, fragrance-free, hypoallergenic, tested eye make-up remover.	Use product with a cotton ball or cotton pad to remove eye make-up. Rinse with tepid water to remove all traces.
Eye treatment: use a cream designed for dry and sensitive skin.	Sweep in from the outer corner of each eye, toward the bridge of the nose, gently applying the cream with your ring finger.
Anti-aging treatment: use a cell-renewal preparation for sensitive skin.	Massage formula into skin on neck, throat, face, and at hairline.

Weekly Care

PRODUCT TO USE	PRODUCT DIRECTIONS
Problem areas: use a clay or drawing-formula mask to lift blackheads and draw out toxins and other impurities. Use peel-off or moisture-conditioning masks to clean deep, lifting away accumulated dead cells.	In summer, spot-mask problem oily areas only. (Not recommended for dry areas.) In winter, spot-mask on dry skin zones only.

Your goal is to be as gentle as possible with your skin. Attend to breakouts or acne eruptions immediately. Your hands and fingertips carry microorganisms that breed on dirt, stale make-up, and polluted oil, so keep hands and fingers off your face.

You must select a treatment system from one cosmetics company. Do not mix treatment products (for example, don't combine cleanser from *X*, toner from *Y*, and moisturizer from *Z*). Fragrance- and oil-free, water-based products that have been tested by dermatologists are recommended.

Here are some do's and don'ts for women with sensitive skin:

☞ Do's

❏ 1. Do drink eight glasses of water daily.

❏ 2. Do use acne-cleansing pads without resorcinol, which is a darkening agent on black skin.

❏ 3. Do stay calm and learn to relax to help chase skin problems away.

❏ 4. Do develop better dietary habits. What you put in your body affects your skin.

❏ 5. Do use special astringent or skin fresheners formulated for sensitive skin.

❏ 6. Do keep your face's dry zones in check.

☞ Don'ts

❏ 1. Don't use astringents designed for oily skin on dry zones of your face.

❏ 2. Don't eat a lot of dairy products, salty and oily foods, or sugar-filled products including chocolates.

Now you know your skin type and have a regimen for daily care. You should, however, take into account the season—spring/summer or fall/winter—when you answer the skin-typing questionnaire. And don't forget to ask yourself if there are any special changes going on: Are you dieting? Do you have your period? Been doing a "lot of partying?" I am sure you know this already, for I mentioned it early on, but it's worth repeating. Since the germinating layer of your skin is fed through your blood system, what you eat and what gets into your blood system has a noticeable effect on your face.

Chapter 4

Facial Hair, Blemishes, and Other Facial Conditions

In this chapter I explain why there are certain skin features such as facial hair, freckles, pimples and blemishes, blackheads and whiteheads, age spots, and so on. If you understand what causes these conditions and know how to cover or remove them effectively and safely, then you will feel better about your face and about your self.

❧ Removing Facial Hair

Hair, particularly facial hair, is a condition many women must address, especially black women. It is not that black women necessarily have more facial or body hair than white women, but the problem has to be approached differently. In beauty salons and clinics, I constantly see black women attacking the hair on their face, underarms, and legs. These women buy product after product at the cosmetic counters in discount drug chains and department stores. Personally, I don't see the hair on women as a problem. But our society has made it a problem. In North America, facial hair is not considered to be a female beauty enhancement or an attractive feature. There are places in the world where men find the hair on women sexy, but this chapter is not for those men or women. Since our society sees hair as a detraction, I deal with it as such here. I concur that when facial hair is a problem—for example, when hair bumps detract from one's appearance or interfere with make-up application—it is an issue to be addressed.

Facial Waxing

Areas of concern are usually the facial hair at the temples, hair at the jawline moving back toward the ear lobe, and hair on the upper lip or chin. More women than you might realize have thick hair growing above their upper lip or on the base of their chin. If you want clear skin, then such hair must be removed, especially if you wish your make-up to have a clear, smooth appearance.

Most white women, especially Nordic women, are fair-skinned and have blonde or sandy-colored hair. They can readily bleach these facial hairs and the hairs appear to fade to become translucent. For most black women, bleaching is not an option. The bleached hair stands out prominently against your dark skin. The only recourse is to have this facial hair professionally removed by waxing. Waxing is a hair removal technique that involves applying a paste of warm wax to the hair surface. The wax is allowed to dry, then it is stripped away. As it is stripped away, so is the hair, leaving the skin beneath smooth. It is painless, and the method can keep the area free of hair for from three to six weeks. Another option is to purchase on over-the-counter hair-removing wax product from a drugstore chain or department store. You can use these products at home, and while the process takes time, you will save money. The home method keeps hairs off for nearly six weeks.

Electrolysis and Depilatrom

Hair can be removed permanently through electrolysis or depilatrom; the latter is a popular new treatment. Sometimes you may experience a degree of sensitivity from depilatrom, but this doesn't last long. Electrolysis, however, can be very costly, since you pay by the number of hairs removed.

Some dermatologists do not recommend electrolysis for black women because many develop scarring around the pores. These areas are damaged and become unsightly after the hairs have been pulled through or by them. Some women build up such scar tissue around the pores that they develop keloids (bumps composed of scar tissue). Black skin, although many-layered, is susceptible to scarring—certainly more so than white skin. Make sure you have a competent electrolysis technician who understands black skin.

There are new gadgets that remove hair electronically, so you can do the procedure at home yourself. Usually such items are sold in the beauty-appliance section of the retail cosmetics outlet or cosmetics counter in better drugstores.

☙ Unruly Eyebrows

Another area of hair growth on the face is the eyebrows. Knowing the technique of shaping the eyebrows is important. A woman is considered lucky if she has eyebrow hairs that lay flat and the eyebrows that are well shaped to complement her eyes. However, most women are not so lucky, and they have to have some hairs removed to get a nice look. Many women prefer not to wear a great deal of eye shadow, but if they do, bushy or unruly hairs springing through the eye shadow and highlighter is unsightly. Others have eyebrow hairs removed because they don't like the way their eyebrows look and can't find a way to manage them. For example, bushy or heavy and coarse eyebrows may require some plucking.

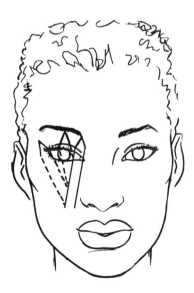

To determine the best length and thickness of your brow, hold the pencil to each nostril and straight up along the nose to the eyebrow. Where it touches the eyebrow is where the brow should begin. Hair between the eyebrows should be removed. Position the pencil vertically over the center of your eye to the beginning of the arch. When you position the pencil from the nose to the outer edge of the eye, you determine the endpoint of the brow and arch.

I find it most unattractive when a woman shaves off her eyebrows and then uses an eyebrow pencil to draw in a line. This gives the face a severe look. Why shave the eyebrow off and then put a new one on, instead of properly shaping or filling in your existing eyebrow?

Nothing is more unsightly than a dramatic, overplucked eyebrow, either. The problem that this may cause—beyond unsightliness—is that when you continually pluck hairs in certain spots, you pull out some of the roots and the hairs will never grow back. Thus you are left with a patchy-looking brow.

Look in the mirror and honestly assess the length and thickness of your brows. If they are bushy and are overpowering your face, then you should remove some hairs. If your eyebrows are too thick and spotty with nicks, then you should shape the brow to complement a natural eyeline. With a brow pencil, you can stroke in between the spaces, filling and shaping the brow. The drawn-on pencil is out of fashion; instead, start from the center of their eye and go upward to the temple, removing from eight to ten hairs.

Tweeze the stray hairs underneath your brow, also. The ideal eyebrow arch is smooth and soft—often referred to as a moon shape. Shape your eyebrow with the peak at the top of your pencil in the center of the brow. To check or correct the shape of your eyebrows, see the illustration on page 53 and at right.

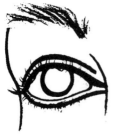

✿ Body Hair

You may want to remove hair from your legs, around the neck, and under your arms. waxing can rid these areas of unwanted hair. There are also depilatories sold in any beauty department that easily whisks away the hair. Let the depilatory set for a few moments and then wipe or rinse hair off with water. Always apply a moisturizer after removing hair from either the face or lower body parts.

✿ Skin Problems

Let's look at the skin "problems" most black women ask me about. Remember, even if you avoid the "don'ts" and do the "do's" in Chapter 3, you may still have skin problems.

Breaking Out

There is no one, specific cause for "breaking out," but it can almost always be stopped or controlled. No matter what the cause, good, regular skin care can help. A healthy regimen plus internal medicine can cure most, if not all, incidents of breaking out and prevent their recurrence.

The type, form, and amount of medicine should be determined by a physician. Obviously, you need not go to the doctor for every blemish. But when you have a blemish that doesn't go away and it bothers you, seek medical advise. Yes, even acne is a condition worthy of a doctor's visit. The person at the cosmetics counter is a beauty adviser, not a physician, even if he or she is a licensed cosmetologist.

The Pill Is Not a Skin Enhancer

Many women have asked me about taking birth-control pills to clear up their skin problems. At this time there is no consensus on the pill's effectiveness in treating skin problem. Research has been done in this area, but at least 25 percent of those studied have seen their skin worsen, and the largest group studied saw no change in skin condition at all. The estrogen in birth-control pills is sometimes used as a skin treatment, but I am opposed to using the pill that way. There are possible side effects from birth-control pills, among them an increase in skin pigmentation and, for some women, the skin gets mottled and darkish.

Menses and Skin Eruptions

Yes, there is an established relationship between your periods and facial eruptions or breakouts. But preventive medication is available. Don't forget, though, that careful cleansing before, during, and after your period definitely helps.

❦ Blemishes

Blemishes are skin faults—for example, blackheads, whiteheads, and pimples. When you see a black head, do you probe and squeeze it? You should not. Squeezing a blackhead can damage the surrounding areas, and you can spread the infection to below the surface, causing other places on your face to erupt. The best way to remove or eliminate blackheads is to keep your skin clean. Remember, you can't have a blackhead without a clogged, oily pore. Therefore, the best approach is super cleanliness—morning and night, and sometimes in between.

The whitehead is so named because the head of the eruption is whitish in color. There are stubborn cases when whiteheads persist, and you should see a doctor or dermatologist, who'll treat it with a miniature scalpel or electric needle. Whiteheads found around the eye (milia) are generally believes to be caused by abrasions or small cuts.

❦ Blotches

To avoid blotches, avoid excessive sunlight. Limit the amount of ultraviolet light that hits your face by using a sunblock, either all over the face or on just the mottled area. Actually, sunblock is a great base for make-up.

If mottled, darkish spots already exist on your face, it is possible to have then removed through dermabrasion—the wearing down of the skin layers until there is clear skin. There are also abrasive scrubs and bleaching creams that can be used directly on the affected area, which help work off the dead, darkened skin.

❧ Wrinkles and Sagging Skin

Wrinkles and sagging skin are due to a breakdown of the skin's collagen, connective tissue, which maintains the skin's elasticity and tightness. Proper skin care not only keeps your skin clear and free of blemishes, but also retards the breaking down of the skin's collagen, reducing wrinkles and sagging skin. Therefore, it is critical that you maintain an adequate collagen level. This can easily be attained by consuming adequate amounts of vitamin C daily. A natural source of vitamin C is rosehips. A rich natural source of vitamins, rosehips contain twenty to forty times more vitamin C than oranges. They also have twenty-five times more vitamin A, 28 percent more calcium, and 25 percent more iron than oranges. Rosehips are extremely rich in Bioflavonoids—co-factors in the vitamin C complex. But whatever you take—natural foods or vitamins—make vitamin C one of your staples, for it is a most important health and facial rejuvenation vitamin.

By utilizing these nutritional tips, you are helping to retard the aging process, collagen breakdown, and maintaining more youthful-looking skin while improving your overall health.

Chapter 5

Coloring Your Skin

The most notable differences among people are their size, features, and color. More often than not, we find the widest variation in size, and so generally we don't classify people by size except to say that they're tall or short, fat or thin. However, we do classify people—rightly or wrongly —by their color and features. Those who are dark-skinned and who have negroid features are perceived to be black whether or not they are. Those who have fair or light "white" skin and aquiline features are more often perceived to be white. These shorthand classifications in many ways are useful, but when you apply them to individuals, they have very little value. When you think in terms of make-up, however, they have value, and that is what this chapter is all about.

❧ Your Facial Skin Color

Melanin is the dark pigment in your epidermis, hair, and eyes that help determine your facial, hair, and eye colors. Melanin and your features determine the colors you should wear. For instance, there are critical differences in applying make-up color to your face. If you are African-American, you must consider all three colors, none of which is neutral. You must look at your hair, eyes, and skin color in determining your make-up color.

Let's start at the beginning. Skin color is determined by three factors: carotene, melanin, and hemoglobin. Carotene gives a yellowish tinge to the skin, while melanin lends a brown color and hemoglobin contributes a reddish hue to the skin. The more melanin, the darker the surface skin tone; carotene, on the other hand, provides contrast with a yellow undertone. The tone and undertone to your skin is based on the amount of carotene and melanin in the epidermis. For example, there are Africans from the Sudan who are so dark that they appear to have a bluish aura to their skin. This is directly related to the amount of epidermal melanin and hemoglobin.

All make-up is created to complement the undertone as well as the surface tone of your face. You may have forgotten the basic color chart, but now you need to know that, in terms of primary colors, brown is really a red. There is a range of colors, or shades, that you should use in your make-up, based on the amount and quality of color in your skin. Although the range of possible colors is wide, it is not limitless. Some colors do not go well with other colors. And the more facial colors you have to work with, the more limited your make-up options. The colors you put on your face should go well with the colors of your hair, eyes, and skin and should appeal to your sense of self as well as be appropriate for the occasion.

Black women today can change their hair color and can appear to have changed their eye color by wearing tinted contact lenses; to some degree, they can even lighten their skin color with bleaching agents or darken it through tanning. But even if you do all this, you will still have three colors to consider.

There are at least 16 million African-American women in the United States, and there are thirty-eight recognized colors of black skin. (White skin has approximately eight to ten skin colors.) So you can readily understand why you need to spend more time understanding color and in choosing color. If you are black, then using make-up colors designed for white skin will probably result in an inappropriate choice. This is because a white woman can apply a much wider range of colors to her face with a less negative effect, since she's starting with a neutral skin color.

❦ Skin Color Classifications

It is popular among cosmetics manufacturers today to classify white skin color by seasons of the year. Those colors that fall within a certain range are called winter colors or fall colors; those that fall within the other range are called summer or spring colors. This may make fashion sense to some, but black skin requires an entirely different classification system.

Among women of color are those who are fair-skinned, with blonde or ash-blond to light-brown hair. Then there are women who have medium-light to dark-brown hair. There are also women with dark-brown to black hair. And finally, there are women with blue-black hair. For example, Trinidadians often have "coal black" hair, which has a bluish cast.

As you can see, we are relating color to color. Skin color bears a relationship to your natural hair color; therefore, I refer to your natural hair, eye, and skin colors in my analysis and charting.

The other feature you need to remember in color coding is your eyes. For blacks, the eye range is from green to hazel, blue to hazel, hazel to light brown, dark brown, and very dark brown. Also, there is a special category for the eye color people from the Caribbean and sometimes Africa have: hazel eyes with a bluish outer rim.

The Fornay Color Chart for Black Women found in the photo insert beginning on page 103 is far more significant for black women, and using it requires far greater care. Make-up for blacks calls for a more delicate balance of colors and shades. Once you know your colors, I'll show you which colors go best together and look best on you. It is hoped that the right color choices go best together and look best on you. It is hoped that the right color choices will make you feel the way you wish to feel and look the way you wish to look.

❧ Color Your Way

If you can remember way back when, you probably once said, "I don't know what colors to wear." Over the years you decided—or someone else decided for you— what colors were best on your face and what colors were best in you wardrobe. Well, maybe you were right and maybe you were wrong.

Be daring enough to go on this color journey with me and see if the colors you chose are indeed your best colors and whether they really please you. Remember: no matter how much a color "may be for you," if you are unhappy with it then it isn't *really* for you. Color not only makes you look a certain way, it makes you feel a certain way as well. And how you feel will affect how you look.

Three Guides, Plus

So far, I have noted the three guides you have in determining what colors to put on your face: your skin tone, your eye color, and your hair color. Those three do not clash with one another. One way or another, they are in harmony, and that is the key. The color you put on your face must harmonize with each feature individually and all three collectively. When this occurs, the invisible fourth guide—the "plus"—comes into play: how you feel and wish to feel.

The Color ABCs

Don' let the myriad of eye shadows, blushers, lipsticks, and nail polishes throw you. There are hundreds of hues but only three basic colors: red, yellow, and blue. This is as important to remember as the fact that black skin generally has one of the following three undertones: yellow, brown, or red-blue, with all their gradations.

You also need to remember that a color will draw from itself. For example, yellow will draw from orange, making the orange look more red. Why does this occur? Since orange is a combination of yellow and red, the yellows are pulled to each other (the yellow in your skin's undertone and the yellow in the color), in a sense leaving the red to stand alone, complementing the yellow.

So, if you have a sallow complexion or a yellow, yellow-red, yellow-beige, or even olive undertone, then red is an inviting color. On the other hand, if you have more of a ruddy complexion, with a more red than yellow undertone, the red draws from the orange, leaving a yellow look. In the same way, if you use green eye shadow and have blue eyes, your eye color drains the blue from the green, leaving a yellow look.

Even though this principle may seem easy, it can get complicated. My color chart in the photo insert takes into account the colors of your hair, skin, and eyes.

There are two factors, however, that the color chart does not address. For these, only you or the situation can determine the best colors. First, some colors make you feel warm, vibrant, and alive, while others make you feel cool, "laid back," and somber. There are sufficient colors in each skin, hair, and eye category to permit you to choose the right color for the mood you want.

Second, certain colors may be more appropriate than others for a particular time of day, occasion, and fashion. You can make the color choices from your category, since each has enough colors from which to select.

Forget the Colors Seasons

You may be surprised that I have not presented colors in terms of seasons of the year. This is because I believe a black woman doesn't need a certain season to wear a given color. She can make herself feel like any season she wants. There is no reason why you can't wear "summer" colors in the winter or "spring" colors in the fall. In fact, you will find any color in nature during any season, someplace in the world.

Likewise, don't get caught by the animal stereotype that colors should be more subdued in the winter and brighter in the summer. This camouflage may help animals protect themselves from predators by allowing them to blend into their surroundings. But you are a proud, lovely black woman who wishes to make a harmonious statement, so make the statement. My color chart helps you make yourself up without either blending into the background or clashing with it. It allows you to be yourself.

❧ Foundations For Your Skin Type

Like many people, you may think of foundation as concealer. But really it's used to impart a hint of color to your skin. Foundation is sometimes referred to as "base," "base color," or "make-up base."

When I talk to African-American women about foundation, I stress that foundation can be used to:

1. Protect against bacteria and impurities.

2. Even out the skin tones—that is, a light T-zone or dark patchy areas.

3. Improve skin texture for a flawless, smooth finish; blushers and other make-up glide on easier and cling better when the skin is covered with a foundation.

4. Kill or decrease sallow skin (a greenish-yellowish or ashy cast), which happens with certain skin pigment types.

5. Create a natural-looking healthy skin glow.

Black cosmetics companies and general-market manufacturers have researched and developed foundations in literally hundreds of forms and shades to meet your every color foundation need. The chart that follows shows the range of foundations available, based on skin type.

Types of Foundations

Skin Type	Formula	Coverage	Texture
☐ Oily (use oil free base)	Liquid/summer Cream/winter Cream to powder/ summer	Light Medium/total Medium	Matte Semi-matte Matte
☐ Dry (use oil-based make-up)	Pancake cream Soufflé cream Stick/tube Liquid	Total Medium/total Total Sheer/medium	Dewy Dewy Dewy Semi-matte
☐ Combination (use water-based make-up)	Liquid Cream to powder Pancake cream	Sheer Medium/total Total	Semi-matte Matte Dewy
☐ Sensitive (use oil-free, fragrance-free tested make-up)	Liquid Cream to powder	Light Medium	Moist Matte

Make-up Finish

Black skin, that looks oily and greasy is not attractive when color is applied. Likewise, dry skin can look dull, sallow, and ashen and will lack a healthy luster without a moist finish. If your skin is very oily and you prefer a finish with no shine or sheen, request a matte make-up finish. If you have normal to combination skin, you may desire an ultra-smooth semi-matte finish (a slight shine). If your skin is dry, strive for a moist dewy finish that will give your skin a natural glow.

During the *extreme hot and humid months* (July and August) in most cities, use three alternatives for relief from very oily skin:

☐ *Clear skin*—light, oil-free moisturizing lotion, with an oil-absorbent, shaded powder.

❏ Use oil control lotion or blotter, with oil control, shaded powder.

❏ *Problem skin*—skip the moisturizing step and apply an oil-free liquid foundation, since the oil from your skin is usually sufficient. Use a deep-pore cleanser and deep-pore cleansing mask frequently, with fragrance-free, dermatology-tested powder shades.

❦ Create Your Specific Foundation Look

When you go to a cosmetics counter, especially one in an upscale department store, it is important to inform the beauty advisor or make-up artist what you are looking for and what you can expect from your foundation make-up. There are some specific foundations that can give you a natural or soft velvet look, or can be a foundation for problem skin that will still give you a soft, natural look.

Create a Bare Healthy Glow Look

Bare healthy glow is a foundation finish that is sheer, light in texture, and provides a natural look. If you have normal to combination skin, then a sheer foundation is usually best. You have nothing to hide and have an even-tone skin.

Create a Velvet Glow Look

Light to medium coverage is the foundation coverage for the woman with an uneven skin tone, with blemishes, or with dull patchy areas and visible pores. When you use velvet glow coverage, the skin takes on a very soft, velvet texture.

Create a Smooth Refined Look

This coverage is perfect when your skin has real problems: stretch marks, dark and light spots, superficial scars, dull sallow places, gray patchy areas, and blemishes. When applied properly, this foundation effect can appear very natural, without a masklike, heavy ashen look. (For best results, consult the facial chart in Chapter 2 for movement directions.)

I do not recommend color washes, bronzing gels, or tints and color adjusters for black women. To date, not enough research has been done on black skin tones to convince me that these items benefit black skin as they do white skin, for which they were designed. I am not against them, but they have not been color-keyed to the thirty-eight shades of black pigmentation.

❦ Your Skin May Need A Concealer

Facial hair is but one skin condition that many women want to alter. Other features you may find disturbing, if not unsightly, are age spots, blemishes, stretch marks, tattoos, birthmarks, varicose veins, and the like.

Before reading the following material and sections you should go back to Chapter I and read the material on nutrition and your skin. But remember that through good nutrition you can improve the health of your skin and thereby erase, retard, or stop some of these detractions. When this is not possible, or in the interim period during improvement, then you can use cosmetic coverings or concealments. But believe me, you can best improve the condition and look of your skin through diet.

"Normal Skin"

What you might call "perfect" skin, we in the cosmetics field call "normal" skin. Normal skin is facial tissue with few blemishes, and very little roughness or peeling. Many of you may have such skin. Normal skin has a uniform coloration that permits the upper skin layer to admit and reflect light (translucency), with unclogged pores. Some individuals maintain their normal skin all their lives with limited effort. But generally they are the exception. For most people, "normal" skin must be achieved—and it is achievable.

Surface Skin is the Key

It will appear that I am repeating myself, and to some degree I am, but surface skin is the key to a fine appearance. And caring for surface skin can improve it. Clearing the surface of dead cells will improve your skin; under normal conditions, it will perfect the condition of your skin.

Clearing should be done with a mild toner. It actually removes the dead skin, which often is not visible to the eye but gives a look of slight roughness and aging. In contrast, when I mention exfoliating, I refer to an astringent, which some women may need.

It Gets Worse Before It Gets Better

If you have neglected your skin—particularly if you have oily skin with subliminal blemishes, blackheads, and whiteheads—your complexion may appear to get worse once you begin taking care of it. You may even find pimples you didn't see before. Don't worry. Your skin is a means by which your body rids itself of impurities. So when you cleanse and improve your system, you may well find your body expelling impurities through its facial pores, and this can result in temporary facial skin problems. Also, what you see on your face may be merely the blemishes becoming more visible as the dead outermost layer is removed. Thus, the blemishes are now closer to the surface and more visible—but also easier to address.

❧ Using a Concealer

If you are working to clear your skin, you'll see progress eventually, but you may want to use a concealer in the meantime. Let's discuss cover sticks (semiconcealers) and concealers themselves in the pages that follow.

Cover Sticks

A cover stick generally comes as a squeezable tube or lipstick-type tube. In either case, you apply the cream to the spot or area you wish to hide. The cover stick is generally for mild pigmentations and discolorations.

Cover sticks are excellent tools borrowed from the theater to spot-conceal flaws anywhere on you face, with special consideration for shadows under the eyes, lines around the eyes near the temple, dark eyelids, lines around the nose and mouth, and the cleft in the chin. Cover sticks usually come in beige-yellow tints in light, medium, and dark and are especially blended for black women. If you have medium-dark skin tone, use a cover stick a shade darker so as not to play up the often lined and puffy tissue. The goal is to give the illusion that where the dark skin, upper lid, and area under the eyes come together is lighter, softer, and therefore, smoother than it really is. In most cases, I prefer to apply the cover stick on top of foundation. The creams blend better and the cover stick formula stays put longer because it has something to cling to; also, it won't crease, slip around, or bleed. Use your ring finger to gently pat on the cover stick formula, as illustrated on page 70. On dry eyelids, use a cover stick to achieve a smoother finish to your eye shadow and to keep the shadow in place. You can also use a cover stick to contour your nose; see the illustration on page 70.

Concealers

Most black women are plagued with scars, pigment discolorations, varicose veins, stretch marks, and the like. The cosmetics industry has finally discovered this and has done an outstanding job in now providing quality products for black women with these conditions. Concealers are waterproof coverups for large areas.

Iman, Flori Roberts and Fashion Fair Cosmetics, respectively, have revolutionized the cosmetics industry with their concealing products keyed to the dark pigmentation of African-Caribbean, African-Latin, African-European, and African-American women—a real breakthrough. Flori Roberts' Derma Blend is especially formulated to cover leg veins and stretch marks. Fashion Fair introduced concealing cream shades called Cover Tone that blend easily with shades in their liquid, cream, and pancake cream foundations. For all skin types, these corrective creams are waterproof, non-greasy, and smudge-free (a plus for oily skin). They easily conceal most skin imperfections, such as scars, burn marks, blotches, blemishes, undereye shadows, age spots, birthmarks, broken capillaries, varicose veins, stretch marks, surgical discolorations, and tattoos. Black women have been waiting for these products for years. I have used both,

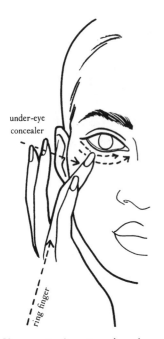

under-eye
concealer

ring finger

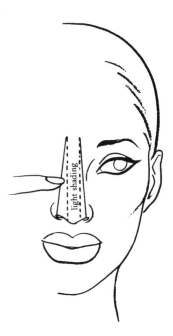

light shading

Use your ring finger to apply under-eye concealer or cover stick beneath the eye or above the eyelid, moving left to right. The cover stick can also serve as a foundation for eye shadow.

Apply light cover stick down the center of your nose. Apply darker cover stick or contour powder on each side of your nose, shading the nostril area. Gently blend with your fingertip and set with powder.

and I recommend them highly. The illustration on page 71 shows how a concealer has been used for vitiligo.

Let's look at the concealer by Fashion Fair. Cover Tone is guaranteed to adhere to your skin when properly applied—so much so that you can go swimming with the concealer on and no one will know.

I will now suggest how to apply a concealer for maximum effect. First, you skin has to be "squeaky clean." The manufacturers supply directions for their products, but they all say basically the same thing: clean skin is a must before application; apply concealer directly to the affected area using a spatula that generally comes with the product; apply the product a little at a time.

If you don't like to use the spatula, use your hands to apply the concealer, but make absolutely sure that both hands are clean. Apply the

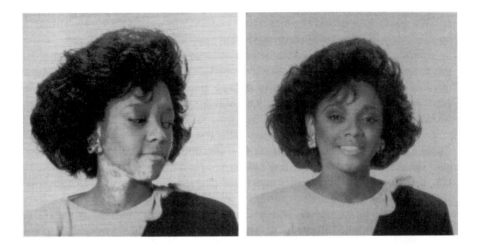

product with your fingertips and gently spread a light covering over the entire area so that the treated area is indistinguishable in color from the surrounding skin. You may find that by warming the product in your hands (the palm), it can be applied easier. Always start at the center of the area and move outward. When the concealer completely covers the area, and is properly matched, it will almost melt and blend into your natural color.

While the concealer is still damp, immediately apply the specially formulated powder in order to set, seal, and dry the concealer. All of this must be done before you can touch the area. It shouldn't take more than a minute to apply the concealer and powder. As long as the concealer is applied rapidly and is still damp when you begin with the powder, you are safe.

Now you can decide whether you wish to use a foundation. Most women will. Apply your foundation along the outer edge of the concealed area. Blend it in there and over the rest of your face.

The key to successful use of a concealer is to pair the right concealer and foundation with your skin color. Then you can blend at the edges, or demarcation line, to achieve a flawless look. For example, Fashion Fair makes a concealer called Brownblaze Glow and a foundation called Brownblaze Glow; these two products should be used together. If the concealer and foundation match your natural skin color, you will have no problem following the directions and getting the required results from Derma Blend, Cover Tone, and Lydia O'Leary products.

❧ Blending Your Foundation

This is a very important step. When I say "blending," that is exactly what I mean: placing the color next to your skin and having it look natural. For example, many women mistakenly apply foundation first to their chin. Instead, they should apply less foundation to the chin so that there is closer harmony with the skin on the neck. You should always blend your foundation downward, with less and less foundation at the chin area. Always blend downward and blend lightly. The downward movement allows for better coverage because of the way facial hairs lie on the skin and hair without streaking.

If you are using a liquid foundation, place four dots of it on your face, then blend them together. (If you have oily skin, and are using an oil-free product, be aware that you must use it rapidly because these products dry quickly—in approximately 30 seconds. If you are too slow, the dots will dry and you will be able to see where you placed them on your face.) The four-dot method is the best approach because you will not use too much foundation, and you will develop a rapid way of getting complete and natural coverage on your face. One mistake many black women make is to put on too much foundation, believing this is the only way to get total coverage. Instead, put one dot on the forehead, one on each cheek, and one on the chin; maybe add one on the tip of the nose (this would be a fifth dot). Use your fingertips and blend the dots into each other, working out to the hairline and jawline.

The best tool for applying a soufflé, cream, or pancake cream foundation is a sponge. I am a firm believer in using a sponge. It is clean and it frees the hands; it is better than your fingertips because the warmth of your fingers can cause streaking. But don't wipe your skin with the sponge. Use a press, dab, and pat movement (see the following illustration). This allows you to place the proper amount of color where it's needed.

As you know, a sponge has holes, and as you press the sponge onto the surface of the foundation, it lifts away the product. So press quickly, lift quickly, and apply to the face. I don't recommend sponges for applying a liquid foundation, though, because they have a tendency to absorb too much liquid. Once you apply the liquid foundation with your fingertips,

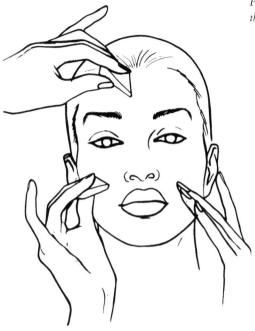

Press, dab, and pat with your fingers, holding the applicator as illustrated. Do not wipe.

however, you can go back over your work with a damp sponge to smooth your foundation to the finish you want.

For those women who use a soufflé with a liquid cream, a cream, or the pancake foundation, the sponge is the best tool for application. The cream stick is another item that can be applied to your face with a sponge.

If you are like many women, you probably use a thick, round sponge that's sold at most cosmetic counters. And if you are like the many women who have spoken to me, you probably find these sponges cumbersome. You have to fold them in half and press them to your skin. Sometimes they unfold, slip, crumble, and even come apart. Why use a big sponge when you use only half—and that half with difficulty? Besides, the round sponge is very difficult to clean. There are square sponges, but most women find them too flat and, again, too cumbersome. The ideal sponge is triangular, so that it can be held between the index and middle finger and the thumb. Use a triangular sponge, employing the technique of press, dab, and pat. Don't wipe, scrub, or use a rubbing motion.

❧ Placing the Foundation on Your Face

Where and how you place the foundation is very important. Once again, think in terms of facial zones. The center zone of your face is called the T-zone, and it is here that you should start to apply the foundation. Begin at the forehead and move toward the temples and around the eye area.

Circle around the eye area as if to get an owl-eye look. You don't want to put foundation on the eyelids or under the eye—just up to the rim of this area. The reason for using this owl-eye approach is that ingredients in some formulations might affect such sensitive areas.

If you have blemishes in these areas, use a cover stick or a concealer as a foundation for eye shadow and to erase any darkness under the eyes. Remember: your application movements should always be outward toward the hairline, but the stroking, pressing, dabbing, and patting motions are lightly downward. This will encourage any facial hair to lie flat, since hair usually grows downward. Movement then is from the center of the T-zone, blending the forehead, temples, and under the eyes, then moving to the cheeks and then lightly from the cheekbone down toward the jawline.

You should lighten your application when reaching the jawline, so that your foundation blends evenly below the jaw. There should be no demarcation line between the jawline and the neck. You do not—and should not—carry the foundation beneath the chin and jawline onto the throat and neck. I repeat: application is from the center of your face outward toward the hairline. The movements are press, dab, and pat, stroking lightly downward to press the hair down.

❧ The Neck Area

For over twenty-five years I have been against putting foundation on the neck; I am still against it, because there is no reason to do it. When the cosmetic chemist keys color to your facial area, he or she uses the color tones in the center of your face, and moves outward toward the hairline to determine your undertone. Colors of black skin vary greatly in terms of shading at the temples, at the center of the face, on the jawline, and on the neck. You can't judge facial color based on the color of your hands, arms, neck or jaw—they are generally all different. So if you want a true facial color tone, you must go by the suggestions I make for matching skin color to proper foundation.

There are but a few exceptions to what I have just stated. If you have an extremely light face, which is much lighter than your neck, then select a foundation that is a little darker, so as to match the dark tones of your neck. If your face is darker and neck lighter, then you should choose a foundation just a little lighter. It may look a little strange at the center of your face when you apply it initially, but as you blend the foundation in, you will see how it complements the neck color.

With this method, your facial color, foundation, and neck color will blend. Remember: when someone looks at you, he or she doesn't stare at your face or neck unless you do something striking to draw the person's eye. What people do, however, is look at you in a general way. You may recall I said at the beginning of this chapter that people look at each other and classify one another. They look for impressions. If you make the areas close to the temples and jawline blend with the neck color, whether darker or lighter than your face, you will convey the impression that both are the same color. It is the eyes' impression that you are after.

Another reason why you should not color your neck is that the cosmetics will soil your clothing. I have found this to be a serious problem for so many women who apply foundation or powder to their necks.

Option: For severe neck discoloration, the smudge-proof/waterproof color coded concealers discussed on page 69 are alternatives.

☙ How To Choose Your Foundation

African-American women choose a foundation that perfectly matches their skin tone (see illustration on page 77). To be able to choose properly, first there are some "don'ts" you should avoid.

❑ 1. Don't try to change your skin tone with foundation. Black models, actresses, entertainers, and opera stars have to change their skin tone for stage effect. However, most women appear in natural light or artificial light. It is important to choose a foundation that coordinates and harmonizes with your skin tone.

☐ 2. Don't buy a foundation without testing several colors in you skin-tone range. Test them in natural and artificial light.

☐ 3. Don't buy one foundation and expect it to impart the right color for four seasons of the year.

☐ 4. Don't wear your friends' foundations. If a friend is in your color range, she might have yellow-olive undertones whereas you might have yellow-red. The foundation will be different, therefore.

☐ 5. Don't rush your purchase. You can't rush into a store on the tail end of your lunch hour and quickly choose the foundation, especially if it's your first time or you have developed new color problems. You must take the time and have the patience to test your foundation, but first check your skin for changes and buy foundation accordingly.

Now that those don'ts are out of the way, here's what you should do. First, because your skin is dark, it is important that you test a foundation based on the season in which it is to be worn. As your skin gets darker or lighter it can take on a golden-red, reddish brown, or brownish blue undertone based on the amount of sun or wind it is exposed to. Don't look for an exact match; you are not involved in true skin-tone matching. For example, in the summer I suggest a summer foundation that cools down the yellow, red, and blue undertones.

A black woman's true skin tone can be tested for accuracy during the latter part of the fall and in the winter months. The situation is different, however, for light, medium, and dark skin tones, for they turn sallow, olive-brown, or deepish yellow-gray or brown. I suggest a winter foundation that imparts golden-beige, copper-brown, and rich red-brown radiance to African skin tones.

Second, you should be aware that there are now fifteen cosmetics companies marketing skin-bleaching agents to black women. These products permit you to even out your skin tone or fade out blotches and superficial spots. The bleaching product blends the shades of the spot and the surrounding skin. These creams also lighten the outer layer, giving an appearance of lighter skin.

When you use these bleaching creams, there is something to remember. Your skin takes on a more yellowish undertone, since you have

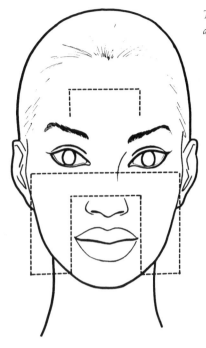

Test the center of your face, cheeks, and jawline to determine a perfect foundation match

bleached out the dark part of the brown pigment in the melanin. This slight difference means you must rematch your foundation.

Third, you should know the effects of your medications. Birth-control pills will darken large parts of your face. Medicine for high blood pressure will sometimes cause the skin to take on a deeper, reddish brown or gray-brown undertones. A liver condition, excessive alcohol consumption, and drug abuse will darken a large section of your face. When such conditions take place, you must revise your foundation. You may have to change the shade until your skin color returns to normal.

Last, make an appointment with a make-up artist or beauty advisor in a retail store or salon. Have the individual do a full-scale make-up application. Refer to our discussion of what you should expect from your make-up, and see the foundation chart on page 65 and color chart on pages 103-110 as well.

Your skin's undertone, as discussed earlier, is the aura or glow of your true skin tone. It can be flushed out by standing in a room or in front of a white wall, with white background, and in natural light. Wrap your hair with your whitest scarf or drape your neck and shoulders with a white sheet. Allow the ultraviolet light to bounce on your face until you can actually see a green (olive), yellow, reddish yellow, reddish brown, or blue aura.

Your Skin Tone and its Undertone

- ☐ *Light skin.* Fair—undertones yellow and olive; light skin—undertones yellow, red, and ruddy.

- ☐ *Medium skin.* Light or medium skin—undertones yellow-sallow; medium skin—undertones yellow to red and ruddy.

- ☐ *Dark skin.* Medium dark skin—undertones golden, brown, and gray; deep dark skin—undertones red, brown, and blue.

Cosmetics Terminology

There are the generic color categories the cosmetics companies use to describe the skin of African-American women. For instance, beige becomes Golden Beige by Company X. Amber becomes Amber Gold by Company Y, and cocoa becomes Cocoa Beige by Company Z. When companies refer to colors in the light-skin category, the generic words are *alabaster, beige, amber, tawny,* and *café au lait.* The cosmetics trade uses the following when describing medium skin: *cinnamon, copper, bronze, light brown.* They refer to the colors of dark skin as *teak, cocoa, dark brown, mahogany.* There are many, many more terms, but these are examples of how the cosmetics industry classifies skin tones and how it tries to give exciting and flattering names to the colors it wants you to buy.

Difficult Matches

For all their research, there is a skin tone that cosmetics companies find difficult to match. It is the tone in the medium range that has yellow or sallow, ruddy undertones. With some searching and patience, however, even this skin tone can be matched to a color foundation.

I have no respect for retail beauty advisors or make-up artists who suggest that a customer mix shades to achieve a match. These are individuals who either don't have the shade themselves, are not knowledgeable, or only want to take your money. If the customer is foolish enough, she will have spent as much as $58 for one shade of foundation to match her skin. Even the wealthy would balk at this price, particularly when the foundation probably costs about $15. There is such a variety of foundations produced for black skin that blending is rarely needed.

☙ Face Powders

Many black women have decided that they do not need or cannot use powder, largely because they have gotten poor results. However, powder can eliminate the shine for those women whose skin tends to be slightly oily.

Applying powder to your foundation also prepares your face, giving it a silky texture on top of which to apply your blush. However, some make-up artists want you to apply foundation first, other colors next, and powder last, to set the face.

Which method you use depends on your skin type. For this decision, I divide black women into two skin types: those with oily skin should apply powder immediately after the foundation; those with dry skin should apply the foundation first, then the eye and cheek color, and set the face with translucent powder.

Types of Powder

There are two types of powder, and they have different purposes beyond that of setting your foundation: translucent setting powders and shaded, or pigmented, powders. Translucent powders are usually loose formulas, with a tint of either amber or bronze. These are usually termed translucent because you can see through the powder to your skin, which will have a glow. These setting powders are used to absorb surface oil and perspiration—for example, for touch ups before work, after lunch, on the T-zone, and on the cheeks.

Shaded powders are for women who prefer to use a moisturizer and may not use a liquid, cream, or pancake cream foundation. They may be bought either loose or solid in a compact. Shaded powder is applied over your moisturizer, and is a pigmented powder.

I have no problem with black women using shaded powders in place of foundation and translucent powder. Remember, though, that pigmented powder not keyed to your foundation coloring can disturb it. For instance, if you have a bronze foundation and you put a sable powder over it, the result will be a muddy look, giving a gray, dull appearance to the skin. In contrast, translucent powders need not match your color skin. They are designed to set the foundation and absorb the perspiration and oil deposits associated with the foundation.

You do not have to worry about today's powders lending an ashy or gray look to your skin. When keyed properly, this will not happen. It is titanium dioxide, a white talcum powder, which usually gives that look to black skin. Just make sure the powder you choose is color right and researched for you. So many black women have had problems in the past, because they used powders designed for white skin, that they now use no powder at all. Fear no more! You can achieve wonderful results with powders that are appropriate for you skin.

In summary, some people want to have moist-looking skin while others want a semi-matte or matte appearance. Powder should be used for the purposes suggested. If you don't want a shine, use powder. The option is yours.

The Benefits of Powder

I have already presented some of the benefits of powder, but now I would like to detail additional ones so that you will know what kind of powder to buy, which brand, and what to avoid. Let's review the already noted benefits of powder:

1. Sets make-up foundation

2. Absorbs oil and perspiration

3. Does away with the shine

In addition, today's powders will not dry your skin. Many black women feel that powder causes a gray or ashy look. This is not true. Most powders have some type of moisturizing agent, and the amount depends on the brand. When properly applied, powders will impart a natural, translucent sheen to the face.

It is important that women with black skin use only translucent powder after applying foundation. You don't want to employ shaded powders to dust or set your foundation. Also, remember that a little powder goes a long way. You don't need to use a lot of powder to set your foundation. A "cakey" effect is not attractive, and it emphasizes any lines you have under you eyes, around the nose and mouth, and even the cleft of the chin. Think of putting a sheer veil over your face; that is the amount of powder to apply. The ideal is to use powder to set the foundation, and to allow the skin and color foundation to glow.

How to Apply Powder

Loose powder comes in a container with a scoop-out feature, so it can be reused and so as not to spoil the entire product. A shaker container is ideal for some women; the powder can actually be shaken out of the container. It is like a salt or pepper shaker, whereby you can measure the amount of powder and control its spillage. There is also a compact powder. In this instance, you cannot shake or pour the powder, but rather, you use a flat puff applicator to lift the powder from the container to your face.

A cotton ball is usually used to apply loose or pressed powder. A powder puff is usually flat and is used for applying pressed powder. The fluffy powder puff is usually used for loose powder, while the fluffy powder brush, which is an ideal applicator, is recommended highly for loose or pressed powder application.

How to Get the Look You Want

What look do you want? The matte look is achieved with loose powder and the fluffy puff. Press, dab, and pat is again the operation in applying loose powder (see illustration on page 82). To achieve a sheen (a moist look), again use loose powder but apply with a powder brush. To achieve an oil-free, perspiration-free look, women with oily skin, or women who do not want a shine in the T-zone, use pressed powder with a flat puff or a cotton ball. Pressed powder, in general, is ideal for oil absorption; in fact, there are pressed powders designed for oil absorption. You should ask for these particular formulas at your cosmetics counter if you are trying to rid your skin of perspiration and oil.

Use a powder puff to press, dab, and pat your face with powder, using downward strokes to encourage any fine hairs to lie smooth and even.

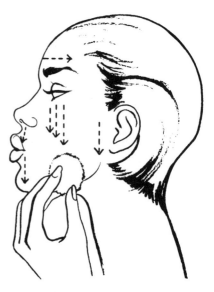

Once again, let's make sure you understand that there should be no scrubbing, no rubbing. To do this only takes off your make-up and redeposits it, usually in the very places you don't want it.

Some Powder Tricks

Use a loose powder whenever you want to take away a line of demarcation. These are usually under the eyes, along the hairline, and on the jawline. Loose powder is excellent for blending your under-eye concealer with your blusher. Setting powder can easily be powdered between these two lines to soften the effect, or even erase it, to become a very natural meeting of color. The trick is to dip the powder brush in the powder and flick away the excess powder, then redip the brush in the loose powder and flip away the loose powder, and then dip the brush into the blusher and shake off the excess. Now you have both the blusher color and the loose powder on the bristles. All you have to do is fan the brush over the line of the demarcation and get a softened effect.

Chapter 6

Coloring Your Face

Now that you have applied your foundation, you are ready to do your eyes, cheeks, and lips. But in order to color your face, you need the proper tools.

☙ Your Color Tools

The tools that I discuss here may, in some instances, be different from those you have previously used. However, these are the ones I believe are the easiest and most functional.

- Powder brush
- Blush brush
- Contour brush
- Eyeliner brush
- Eye shadow sponge
- Eye shadow brush
- Brow brush
- Lash comb
- Lip liner pencil
- Lipstick brush

The right equipment is important, but you also must know the proper techniques and procedures. Your make-up steps now come into full use. In the previous chapters we discussed skin care, foundations, and powders. Now is the time you begin to apply what you have learned. I know that many of you will have your own techniques and procedures already, but I urge you to compare your methods with what I am about to propose. And for those of you who have no method, or who have been confused by the myriad of products put in front of you, I offer the following steps:

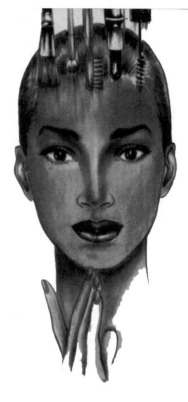

1. Cleanse

2. Tone

3. Moisturize

4. Apply concealer
   (this is optional; I suggest either Flori Roberts' Derma Blend, Fashion Fair's Cover Tone, or Lydia O'Lery's concealer)

5. Apply foundation, or base

6. Apply concealer (this is optional)

7. Contour the cheeks

8. Apply powder

After the above steps, you might want to apply eye make-up (see page 87). Next, apply blusher and then lipstick. Some women prefer a different order; they might go to the blusher, then to the eyes, and then do the lips. The choice is yours.

☞ Your Eyes and the Use of Color

When I think of eyes, I think of Erykah Badu, Brandy, Regina, Vivica Fox, Lena Horne, Tyra Banks, Pam Grier, Angela Bassett, Vanessa Williams, Naomi Sims, Beverly Johnson, Nancy Wilson, and Barbara Smith (model and restauranteur)—all with eyes that allure, that hold, capture, and hypnotize you.

These are the faces of visible African-American women, and their eyes are made up to hold our attention. Because of this, many black women tend to admire and sometimes yearn to look like these women. I understand this but I disagree. These beautiful women are made up for the world of films, entertainment, and fashion. They do not live your lifestyle.

I have had the privilege of designing the eye color for models such as Wanakee, Iman, and Beverly Johnson, and singers Nancy Wilson, Gladys Knight, Melba Moore, and Natalie Cole. The eyes of these women are beautiful, and after the eye statement they are more beautiful, but the look of each is individual, suited to that person and the world in which she works.

Religion and Color

The celebrities I just named are images of a world far from the one that most black women know and live in. The facts are, as stated earlier in this book, that the majority of black women do not wear color make-up, or wear only very little. Probably as many as sixty-five percent do not wear those wonderful and exciting eye colors and blushes.

There are reasons for this situation. Regardless of where they live now, most African-Americans came from the South. Many who live in Detroit, Chicago, Philadelphia, Washington, DC, New York, or Newark have families who came north through "the corridor" during the great migration. And many first-, second-, and third-generation "Northerners" still hold very tightly to their conservative religious and southern cultural roots. The church in the South, and also in many major northern cities, is the central institution for blacks, next to the family. It is where they congregate for religious, social, and psychological security. The religious background of African-Caribbeans, and people of African ancestry in England and Canada, is not unlike that of African-Americans. The culture of these blacks is also steeped in religion and has certain notions of what a "good" woman is.

The church taught that, Only the harlot in the brothel wore color and painted her fingers and toes. So that took care of that! For a time the attitudes extended also to women who went into the theater and other fields of entertainment. These occupations meant you had to "paint" your face and supposedly you lived a "fast" life. Well, these teachings stuck. As strange as it may seem, black men accepted them as much as did women. So, today there may be two forces working against a black woman's wearing of color: these past religious ideas and a boyfriend or husband who wants to see his wife "pure."

Times Are Changing

Times are indeed changing, but attitudes and beliefs die hard. The vast majority of black women are still churchgoers, particularly women in the South. So the idea of putting on color is slow to be accepted; when it is, the color goes on subtly and with a look of total naturalness. In many instances foundation is the only color. So this is where we begin and on what we build.

If you are one of these hesitant women, there are role models more appropriate for both your beliefs and your lifestyle than Tyra Banks or Angela Bassett. For instance, there are such models as the TV star Sheryl Lee Ralph, whose eyes are never overly made up. She is made up to represent what the black professional woman, who is also a mother, can and should look like. There is a naturalness to her fully made-up face, and her eyes never have excessive color, yet she looks lovely.

There are appropriate models for professional women. For example, look at Dr. Mae Jamison, the first black female astronaut, and take a look at the African-American wives of the black mayors of major cities; watch the wives of our black fire and police commissioners. See the black wives of football or basketball stars. Look at professional women athletes, too. They have all done an excellent job. The African-American women who are presidents of black colleges or presidents of major black organizations—they all make excellent role models. They are never overly made up; they never have too much make-up on their eyes.

In fact, too much make-up up on dark eyelids is unattractive. Never overdo your eyes. Look at how attractive the women just mentioned are. That is because everything blends and nothing seen in daylight is overstated. **Keep the sparkle and pizzazz for special evening affairs.**

Refined, secure black women show themselves by making a clear, natural, never overcolored statement to the world. They dress and use color based on the occasion. As a black women, you are about serious business. You are striving to be the best you can—at work, in your social affairs, at home, and in church. You should achieve notice through the quality of your performance, not through garish make-up or inappropriate use of color. Now, let's begin to dress your eyes with appropriate color.

❧ How to Apply Eye Make-up

I have designed a simple system for you. It is a four-step, full-scale rainbow eye system in which we consider the correct approach to the eye shape, eyeliner, and lash application. The color chart in the photo insert on pages 103-110 will guide you in making appropriate color choices. The major principle is to keep the look clean, blended, and subtle. The exception is with evening make-up, when you should exaggerate to shine and sparkle, when *pizzazz* is the operative word. Here is the order for applying eye make-up:

1. Eyeliner

2. Eye shadow

3. Mascara

4. Eyebrow make-up

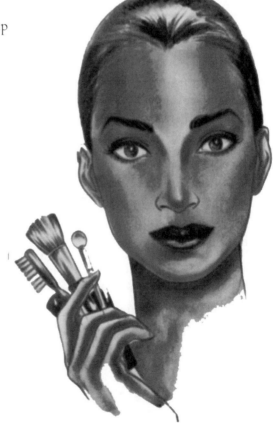

❧ Eyeliner

Eyeliners come in formulas designed for each skin type and in different forms: soft pencil, liquid, cream, and pressed cake.

Eyeliners are used to give more definition to the eyes. They highlight the eyes and make the eyelashes appear fuller and thicker. A person can really bring the desired effect to the eyes with a liner; it is the ultimate groomer because it separates the shadow from the lashes via a circle around the eyes.

I think a smoldering and smoky look around the eyes is most attractive on black women, especially darker-skinned women. Eyeliners to some degree have been in disfavor recently because of how they are sometimes worn, giving the eyes a thick and harsh look. But now there are many shades in complementary neutral tones. Rich, deep blues look exceptionally well on black women with medium to dark skin tones. When you use the eyeliner, be sure to color the top lid as well as the bottom.

There is a technique I would like to suggest, especially to those who have problems finding an eyeliner to complement your various shades of eye shadow or your pupils. Take your eye shadow color—maybe the corresponding shade in a dual kit—and simply wet your brush, then stroke the cake of eye shadow for your eyeliner color. For example, if for evening wear you want to use a reddish eye shadow close to the lash, with a dominant red eyeliner that has a little gold in it, moisten your brush and then stroke with the golden-red eye shadow; draw in the color and, presto, you have an eyeliner in a corresponding shade.

Pencil vs. Liquid Eyeliners

Liquid eyeliner is still one of the most popular forms, but I recommend the pencil eyeliner because you can control it better. Pencils come in more colors, they can be smudged on the top and bottom of the eyelids; and they can be applied either thick or thin. If you have had very little practice applying liquid eyeliner, you can easily lose control. Yet both forms are serviceable and can have attractive results.

Purchasing Your Eyeliner

The eyeliner should be color coordinated with your eye shadow. Eyeliners, especially pencils, can be tested at the cosmetics counter. Testing foundations as well as eye, cheek, and lip colors is permitted in department stores, chain stores, and some pharmacies. And you should test the colors. Try to test them in natural light, even if you have to stroke the color on your face or eyelid and then excuse yourself to walk to where there is natural light. Use your make-up mirror to look at the color on your skin, and you will see that in different lighting the shades appear differently.

Just two words of caution. There are waterproof eyeliners that tend to be a little rubbery, but they are excellent if you perspire heavily, if your skin is oily, or if you go swimming a lot. However, I have found that when used frequently these waterproof eyeliners can actually dry out the area around your eyes, leaving it sensitive. This is especially true for those who suffer from allergies or who are naturally sensitive in this area. If this is your situation, then I suggest you avoid the waterproof eyeliners.

Eye Shadow

Eye shadow comes in cream, crayon, powder, or liquid. The powder shadows are ideal for most skin types because they can be controlled easily and they appear to be softer, silkier, and smoother on your skin. However, the powders are best suited for oily, combination, and normal to oily skin.

The cream shadows are best for women with very dry eyelids. The only caution is that women with medium to dark skin tones stay away from creams that have a silver or white talc base, since these shadows give the eye area an ashen look. The light materials play up the gritty, chafed areas and dry lines of your eyelids.

The crayon shadows are excellent for smoothing on and blending in. They can be very soft, and that is the caution for those of you who have oily skin. Make sure you don't overuse an oil-based crayon shadow, for it can build up a crease and melt on the eyelids.

There are several cosmetics companies that encourage customers to dampen their powder eye shadows because it gives it a different consistency

Basic eye color application

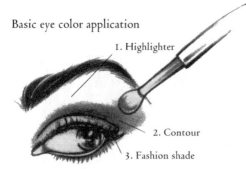

1. Highlighter
2. Contour
3. Fashion shade

A. For a basic eye color effect, apply highlighter, contour, and then fashion shade.

Multicolored eye

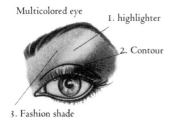

1. highlighter
2. Contour
3. Fashion shade

B. For a rainbow, multicolored effect, apply highlighter, contour, and then the fashion eye color.

A. To make your eyes less round:
Liner
Draw a thin line at just the very outer corner of the upper lid and across the bottom lid.
Shadow
Use lots of color, edging shades into the contour crease, shading up and out at the corner.

B. To make eyes more prominent:
Liner
Draw a line from the center of the upper lid out toward the corner. Add a line across the bottom lid.
Shadow
Add a light color to the eyebone, contour color in crease, and use a frosted or light shade on the lid.

C. To make eyes look deeper:
Liner
Draw eyeliner across the top lid and from the center to the outer corner. Apply mascara.
Shadow
Add lots of color in the contour crease. Do not apply light frosted shades.

D. To make small eyes look larger:
Liner
Circle the top and bottom inner lids with soft black, deep blue, or rich deep brown; all three colors will make the white of the eyes appear even whiter and the eyes appear wider. Apply mascara.
Shadow
Color is applied to the eyebone under the brow arch, fanning out toward the temples. Contour color in crease and along the lid as illustrated.

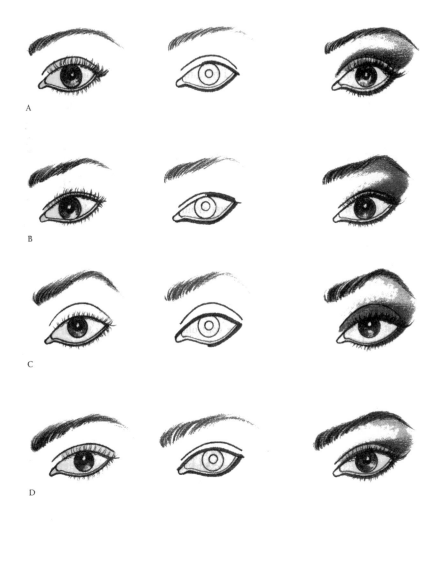

and helps them glide on evenly, dry well, and stay put. One such company is Fashion Fair. Its instructions ask you to moisten the eye shadow in its dual kit with an eye shadow brush or sponge, and to stroke the eye shadow onto the eyelid so it will dry to a very soft color. The color remains true and stays put, without the creasing so often seen when a cream or liquid shadow is used. The technique is excellent for oily skin.

There are fragrance-free eye shadows, produced by companies such as Aveda, for those of you who have sensitive eyes or tend to have an allergy-prone eye area.

There are eye shadows that are sold as dual kits: two pans containing two colors that usually are a highlighter and a fashion shade, which can also be used for contours. Then there are four-pan color kits: highlighter, contour, and a fashion shade in a light and a dark hue. You can even find six- and twelve-color pan kits that permit you to mix and blend shades to come up with original colors for a rainbow eye, smoldering eye, or contour eye.

Highlighters do not have to be eggshell white or creamy white. They can be pink or dark lavender, or a light shade of blue or even a dark shade of blue. The highlighter you use depends on the effect you want. Again, experiment to come up with original ideas, but consult the color chart in the photo insert for the right colors.

Contour shades usually come in neutral colors like cocoa or light brown, or in shades of gray and in the berry shades.

❧ Mascara

The purpose of mascara is to build up your lashes. Mascara makes your lashes look longer, thicker, and more smoldering. There is a formulation that comes as a cream, which I recommend. For application, see the following illustration.

The shades that look best on black women are black, brown/black, dark brown, antique bronze, and berry shades, the newest entries on the market. Don't be turned off by the color intensity in the tube. When applied, these berry shades look very soft around the eyes. In fact, the raspberry, cranberry, green, and navy blue shades look fabulous, day or night.

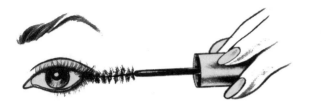

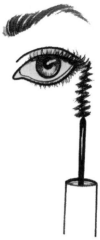

For women with semistraight lashes, hold the brush horizontally and do entire lash, outward and upward, rolling the wand for fullness.

For women with very curly eye lashes, apply mascara vertically. Move from left to right and hit only the tips of the lashes.

Don't be reluctant to try colorful mascara. Many white women are discouraged from using these colors during the day, but on professional black women they look excellent anytime. They give a soft and handsome look to the eyes. Pay attention to your mix of colors when you make up, though. Be careful what color eye shadow you use with a colored mascara. There should be some coordination of colors between the lashes and the eyelid itself.

Remember to test the mascara before you buy, but don't allow the beauty adviser to apply it from the tester wand directly to your eyelashes. This tester wand has been used on other women, and any bacteria it picked up from them is in the tube. Bacteria grow extremely fast in the dark warm tubes on the lighted cosmetics counter. That tester wand could put bacteria on your eyes, so make sure you get a clean wand. Cosmetics companies provide disposable wands for testing purposes.

❦ Eyebrow Make-up

Blessed is the woman who does not have gaps and scars in her eyebrows. She does not need make-up. If you are one of these women, then all you have to do is groom and shape your eyebrows with a brush. However, for most women eyebrow make-up fills in the spaces between the hairs and covers any scarring in the brow area.

Eyebrows can easily be filled in with a pencil to give more definition to the line. But don't think in terms of starting at the beginning of your brow and drawing a line to the end, out toward the temples. This is shaping the brow, and in Chapter 4 there is an explanation of how to shape the eyebrow with tweezing. Now you'll just be filling in the spaces between the hair, according to the existing shape. See the following illustration for instructions on filling in sparse eyebrows.

Eyebrow make-up can also be used where you have overtweezed or overplucked. Shape the eyebrow with the pencil and fill in until new growth appears, then do your reshaping. Also, don't be afraid to experiment with the eyebrow. Some eyebrows look great brushed straight up, toward the hairline; just brush them up and fan them out toward the temples. This is a great look, especially for evening.

For sparse eyebrows, fill in spaces, moving from inner corner of the eyebrow outward.

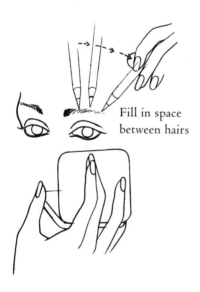

Fill in space
between hairs

✤ Blushers

The purpose of a blusher is to bring a blush and glow to the cheeks. I recommend using blushers because they bring a vibrancy and alive quality to your face. But you must carefully select the color and place it correctly.

Don't be dissuaded from using blusher because you see intense color compacts on display at retail cosmetics counters. They are usually very bright or very intense, but you will be surprised how, when keyed to your skin color, those deep, rich pigmented blushers bring a soft natural glow to your cheeks.

You have probably heard the cosmetics trade call their blusher colors Mahogany, Golden Bronze, Loganberry, Raspberry, Topaz, Ruby, Ginger, Gold, Cinnamon, and Brown. These are the names of just a few of the blusher products produced. Black companies recently have developed many natural, warm, and sophisticated deep-pigmented shades for black skin, which have proved to be excellent.

Your lipstick and blusher do not have to match; however, they should be of the same color family or in the same color range. For example, a red-brown blusher enhances a yellow-based red lipstick. For evening, a true red blusher with golden highlights makes a wonderful partner to a gold-frosted red lipstick with a golden gloss. With this combination your cheeks and lips will be all aglow with golden sparkle, reflecting light against your dark skin. Consult the color chart in the photo insert for more blusher-lipstick combinations.

There are many kinds of blushers sold, with different effects and for different skin types. See the chart on page 97 for information on each. Here, I discuss two major types: powders and creams.

Powder Blushers

Powder imparts a natural-looking, soft-matte finish. Of all the formulas, it is the easiest to apply and looks the best on black skin. Powders glide on smoothly and don't leave a bumpy, ashen buildup. Literally hundreds of powder blushers are available, tailored for every skin type. If you try a blusher that gives a gray appearance to your skin, you can be sure it was not designed for your skin coloring. All skin types can wear powder blusher; however, they are best for those with combination or oily skin. Women with sensitive skin must be very careful, and only use blushers designed for sensitive skin (usually fragrance- and oil-free formulas).

Cream Blushers

There are two basic cream blushers—regular and oil-free—and they come as a swivel stick or in a compact. Use your fingers or the swivel stick for best application. Apply the cream over your foundation and then add your translucent powder. In general, cream blushers are easy to blend, but avoid the pale shades, red to pinks, and peachy to orange colors, because they appear to be suspended in air or to sit on top of the skin.

Cream blushers are best for combination or dry skin. Oily skin collects the shine and high humidity, and in summer months the cheeks appear greasy and slick—not attractive at all! All skin types should stay away from the frosted cream blushers unless the frost is gold, not silver. I don't think silver enhances medium to dark complexions and it should never be used on the cheeks.

❧ Make-up Your Way

Make the Most of Make-up

Here are some new recommendations for your consideration:

❑ Dark & Lovely Cosmetics

❑ Aubarale Skin Care & Make-up Cosmetics
(513) 874-1700, Fax: (513) 874-1700

❑ Sacha Cosmetics Limited of Trinidad
(809) 673-1091, Fax: (809) 673-1029

A fabulous new, well-researched and innovative line, Interface, makes it's entry in major department stores this year. Patricia French's Gazelle line, Iman, Fashion Fair, and Flori Roberts still hold the largest range of foundation colors and continue to advance in research and development.

Here's a list of cosmetic lines that cater to broader markets, especially women of color:

❑ Bobbi Brown: Great color selections and skin care.

❑ Stila Cosmetics: Specializes in eye shadow and lip color.

❑ Francois Nars: Developing more appropriate hues and tones for women of color.

Types of Blushers

Type of Blusher	Finish	Coverage	Type of Skin	How to Apply
Gel tint	Smooth sheen, gold-frosted gels look great at night; don't ever wear frost during the day	Sheer, light texture; should not be deeply pigmented	Combination to oily (most are oil-free and water-based); not advised for very dry skin; can appear shiny and slick	Use fingertips, on top of foundation, before powder; dry-down period is extremely fast, so you have to work quickly; gel can streak and blotch
Liquid	Moist and smooth	Sheer, light to medium texture; deeply pigmented	All skin types; best suited for combination, medium to dry skin	Use sponge, sliding on top of foundation, then set with powder; easy to apply
Mousse	Soft, dewy-looking; gold-frosted is good at night	Sheer, foam is light textured; not deeply pigmented	Not for dry skin; for oily or combination skin	Use fingertips; blend with a sponge, especially around the edges
Cream	Smooth, dewy; gold-frosted is excellent, some even appropriate for day; best for evening wear, and silver-frosted is out forever!	Medium; deeply pigmented; should not ever appear greasy or slick	Normal to dry skin; oil-free best suited for oily only	Use fingertips and blend on top of foundation, set with powder
Powder	Matte or semi-matte frost; gold-frosted is best to highlight cheekbones at night	Medium; deeply pigmented	All skin types; oily skin benefits the most	Use brush; see illustration on page 99

Use Blushers with Moderation

Many women wear too much blusher during the day. The ideal application is only a suggestion, or hint, of color. Select rich, pure colors such as copper-bronze with its deep gold base, or a soft plum, light wine-burgundy, or deeply pigmented almond orange shade. When you apply powder blusher, always dip the brush quickly and flick or twist your wrist to stroke the cheek lightly. Remember: it is better to apply just a little blusher and then go back and apply more if you need it, than to apply too much and have to disturb the foundation to remove the excess. Matte colors (no shine) are best for day on all skin types. For the evening, gold essence, frosty, and shimmery shades are best.

Generally, I don't recommend stripping, or streaking, even though it is very popular. However, in the evening for dramatic effect, it might work rather well. Stripping is a theater technique transferred to retail cosmetics. The aim is to have the skin look as though it had been drenched or kissed by the sun, and the effect is achieved by streaking the color at the temples, cheeks, tip of the nose, and chin. Usually it doesn't work. You have to be very good and have a very light touch. It works best, if at all, on white skin. And unless you live in California, Florida, or another sunny climate, it won't look real.

Color Placement

The cheek, according to your facial shape and size, is where you should place the blusher. Don't place it on the nose. After all, why put blusher where it will make you look like you have a cold?

The outer corner of your eye is your guideline for application. See the following illustration. Don't ever bring the color toward the broad nostril of your nose; it will ring and broaden your facial structure. Like-wise, blusher should not ever be shaded down past the tip of your nose. Draw an imaginary line from the tip of your nose, under your natural cheekbone, to the middle part of your ear; this is usually where you should cut off the shading. Also, most women have a convex eye area, so don't bring the blusher too close to the outer eyes. When applied close to the eyes blushers tend to make them look puffy and drawn.

Consult the color chart on pages 103-110 and the application illustrations that follow, and the recommendations of the cosmetic company. We have included a work sheet for your personal blusher application in Appendix I.

Blushers can do more to add warmth and radiance than any other cosmetics We feature the following four basic face shapes; however, different faces require different techniques. If your face shape is not here, combine the features from others to obtain the right techniques.

To find your face shape, tie your hair up and away from your face and look into the mirror. If you still can't tell, get a ruler and measure your forehead from temple to temple, cheekbone to cheekbone and jawline to jawline. Place measurements on paper and connect with rounded lines.

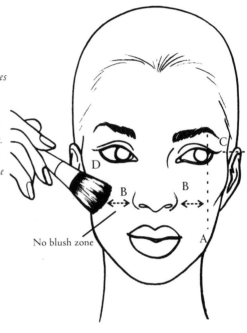

No blush zone

SPECIAL TIPS:

1. *Use the outer corner (A) as a guide to start adding blusher*

2. *Never apply blusher in the No Blush Zone (B).*

3. *Always move across, upward, and out toward the hairline (C).*

4. *Do not add blusher underneath the eyes near the lower rim (D).*

Contouring or shading your facial features is the easiest way to slim down the face and redefine flawed features.

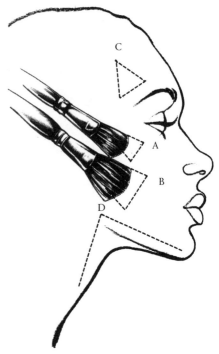

A. *On the top side, apply the radiant, vibrant blusher with your brush sweeping across the cheekbone, blending upward to top of the ear.*

B. *Use your contour brush and apply a rich matte brown on the bottom side of your cheekbone, moving toward the center Part of your ear upward.*

C. *For that special glow at night, apply flesh golden powder blusher on temples, between the eyes, on tip of nose, and at base of chin.*

D. *Use your contour brush to de-emphasize a full or square chin with a matte brown blusher.*

Special Blusher Tips

For the ultimate, long-lasting glow, apply a cream blusher over your foundation and set it with translucent powder. Then apply a complementary powder blusher over the translucent face powder and blend. You will have a day-long natural glow.

SQUARE FACE:

You have a firm structure, usually a wide forehead, cheeks, and jawline. The apple, or round part of the cheekbone, registers near the outer corner of your eye. Begin the blusher application at this point, sweeping the cheek color wide upward to the center part of the ear.

To soften a wide and square face, apply cheek color at the bottom side of the jaw, with the cheekbone to accent the center of your face. Don't ever apply blusher between the No Blush Zone apple of the cheekbone and the bloom of the nostril. Your eyebrows are most important. No straight thin lines. Arch your brows at the outer corner of the pupil, looking straight into the mirror, so they are in line with your cheekbones.

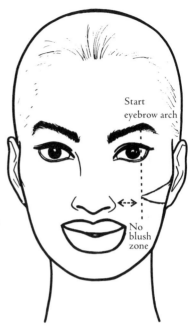

Start
eyebrow arch

No
blush
zone

ROUND FACE:

You have a solid structured face. Keep color high on the cheekbone, sweeping it outward and upward to the top of the ear and hairline. Don't ever place color on the apple and never bring color from the apple toward the bloom of the nostril.

You want to discourage a clownish appearance. Keep color high on the top side of the cheekbone. Sweep blusher from the outer corner of the eye, fanning upward. Eyebrows should be naturally full and shaped horizontally with a slight curve. The rainbow eye placed diagonally plays down circles. Shading is appropriate at the temples. The eyes are the facial point: keep lip pencil line faint and inside the natural lip line.

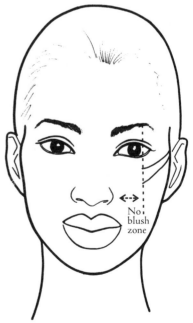

No
blush
zone

OVAL FACE:

*You have the so-called balanced facial structure.
Polish the cheekbone with rich, radiant color, sweeping
from the outer edge of the corner of your eye and
cresting for a V effect. The open part of the V spreads
wide toward the ear and hairline.*

*Play up the apple, moving straight across and fanning
outward. Eyebrows take on a subtle half-moon shape.
Accentuate the crease and create a more concave
illusion. Highlight with greasy mascara. Place
shading color at the temples, on tip of the nose, and at
chin. Lips are shaped, moist, and dewy.*

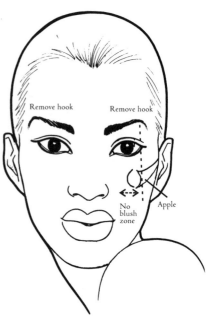

NARROW FACE:

*You have a slim, delicate structure. Start your blusher
placement at the outer edge of the apple. Keep color on the
cheekbone toward the top. Make wide sweeps toward the
upper part of ear and hairline.*

*You want to create optical and aesthetic horizontal lines of
color to suggest width. Don't shade or contour the temples,
jawline, or chin. Color in the center zone of the face is
important. Eyebrows should be on a horizontal plane, with
a high center arch. Eye shadow is earthy, gold, topaz,
peachy-red, soft berry; no brown-black or black outer
corner shading. Lip pencil liner emphasizes, broadens, and
plays up full lips. Apply color to the very edge.*

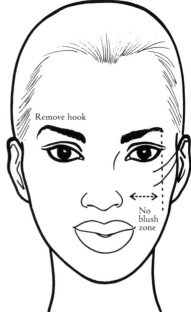

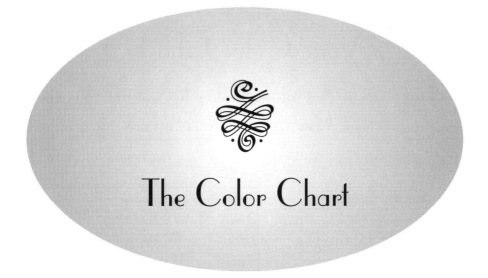

The Color Chart

The Color Chart presents most skin, eye, and hair color combinations. Find your combination of colors on the chart and move horizontally to the far right for the colors best suited to you. If your color combination isn't on the chart, choose the color mix closest to yours, then take only those colors which are the same in all three categories: these are your colors. With this chart, I give you makeovers and examples that will help you use the Fornay Color Chart for Black Women.

Once you have used the color chart and have found your colors, decide which you wish to wear based on your mood and the occasion. Remember to exploit color. When using a color like gray, be bold. Try various shades of gray, from those with a lot of white in them to others of the boldest black. Do the same with your greens and reds.

Your Color Chart

Best Cosmetic & Fashion Colors to Select for Your Skin, Hair, Eyes, and Total Look

Skin Color/Undertone	Hair Colors
Light Skin/Yellow Undertone	*Light Skin/Yellow Undertone*
Red ▦ Violet ▦ Blue Green ☐	Black ▦ Red ▦ Blue ▦
Red Orange ▦ Blue Violet ▦	Green Violet ▦ Blue Violet ▦
Burnt Amber ▦ Yellow Ochre ☐	Red Violet ▦ Burnt Sienna ▦
Burnt Sienna ▦ Thalo Green ▦	Orange Crimson ▦ Black ▦
Burnt Umber ▦	Brown ▦ Burnt Umber ▦
	Violet ▦ Crimson ▦ Orange ▦
Light Skin/Yellow Red (Ruddy)	*Ash Blond*
Bluish Brown ▦ Bluish Gray ▦	Bronze ▦ Blue ☐ Violet ▦
Blue Violet ☐ Blue ▦ Green ▦	Blue Violet ▦ Wine ▦ Green ▦
Violet ▦ Emerald Green ▦	Burnt Sienna ▦ Black ▦
Blue Green ☐ Bronze ▦	Pale Red ▦ Pink ▦ Red ▦
Black ▦ Crimson ▦	Emerald Green ▦
Light Skin/Yellow Beige	*Ash Blond/Light Brown*
Cadmium Yellow ☐	Deep Golden Blond ▦
Pale Thalo Green ▦ White ☐	Light Brown ▦ Deep Honey Blond ▦
Burnt Sienna ▦ Orange ▦	Ultra Mauve ▦ Blue ▦
Crimson ▦ Ultra Mauve ▦	Emerald Green ▦ Pale Green ☐
Blue ▦ Thalo Green ▦ Gray ▦	Dark Green ▦ Black ▦ Orange ▦
Charcoal Gray Blue ▦	Crimson ▦

Your Color Chart

Best Cosmetic & Fashion Colors to Select for Your Skin, Hair, Eyes, and Total Look

Eye Color	Best Cosmetic & Fashion Colors for Your Total Look
Green Brown ▢ White ▢ Cadmium Blue ▢ Yellow ▢ Light Burnt Umber ▢ Cadmium Orange ▢ Orange ▢ Black ▢ Red Violet ▢ Violet ▢	Red ▢ Violet ▢ Blue ▢ Orange ▢ Green ▢ Burnt Umber ▢ Blue Violet ▢ Black ▢
Blue/Hazel Rose ▢ Copper ▢ Deep Burgundy ▢ Blue Violet ▢ Deep Blue ▢ Green Blue ▢ Pine Green ▢ Olive Green ▢ Blue ▢ Gray ▢ Bluish Brown ▢ Green ▢ Emerald Green ▢	Blue ▢ Blue Violet ▢ Green ▢ Red ▢ Pink ▢ Black ▢ Emerald Green ▢
Green/Hazel Green ▢ Blue Green ▢ Blue ▢ Gold ▢ Light Brown ▢ Violet Gray ▢ Slate Gray ▢ Deep Red ▢ Deep Blue Green ▢ Red Gold ▢ Cadmium Yellow ▢ Pale Green ▢ Orange ▢ Burnt Sienna ▢	Green ▢ Orange ▢ Ultra Mauve ▢ Blue ▢ Light Brown ▢

Your Color Chart

Best Cosmetic & Fashion Colors to Select for Your Skin, Hair, Eyes, and Total Look

Skin Color/Undertone	Hair Colors
Light Skin/Medium Olive	*Medium Light/Medium Brown*
Reddish Brown ▦ Violet ▦ Gray ▦ Green ▦ Yellow ▦ Red ▦ Blue ▦ Blue Green ▦ Emerald Green ▦	Gold ▦ Soft Bronze ▦ Blue ▦ Green ▦ Yellow ▦ Pale Green ▦ Deep Green ▦ Crimson ▦ Orange ▦ Charcoal Gray ▦
Medium Skin/Light Brown	*Medium Brown*
Orange ▦ Ochre ▦ Green ▦ Black ▦ Crimson ▦ Burnt Sienna ▦ Blue ▦ Yellow ▦ Red ▦	Medium Bronze ▦ Deep Bronze ▦ Pink ▦ Yellow ▦ Gray ▦ Black ▦ Light Yellow ▦ Green ▦ Red ▦ Crimson ▦
Medium Skin/Brown	*Brown*
Green ▦ Russet ▦ Pink ▦ Mauve ▦ Deep Green ▦ Blue ▦ Green Violet ▦ Red Violet ▦ Gold ▦ White ▦ Red Brown ▦ Orange ▦ Yellow Ochre ▦	Deep Bronze ▦ Orange ▦ Pale Green ▦ Yellow Ochre ▦ Ultra Mauve ▦ Blue ▦ Orange ▦ Crimson ▦ Emerald Green ▦ Deep Red ▦ Pink ▦

Your Color Chart

Best Cosmetic & Fashion Colors to Select for Your Skin, Hair, Eyes, and Total Look

Eye Color	Best Cosmetic & Fashion Colors for Your Total Look
Hazel/Golden Brown Green ▢ Yellow ▢ Red Violet ▢ Blue ▢ Copper Gold ▢ Deep Blue ▢ Deep Green ▢ Mauve ▢ Reddish Brown ▢ Gray ▢ Emerald Green ▢	Yellow ▢ Blue ▢ Green ▢ Gray ▢ Gold ▢
Hazel/Light Brown Black ▢ Deep Brown ▢ Gray ▢ Green ▢ Red ▢ Deep Blue ▢ Deep Green ▢ Mauve ▢ Yellow ▢	Green ▢ Black ▢ Blue ▢ Red ▢ Gray ▢
Light Brown/Gray Deep Red ▢ Medium Pink ▢ Blue Violet ▢ Fawn ▢ Yellow Ochre ▢ Pale Green ▢ Burnt Sienna ▢ Crimson ▢ Orange ▢ Pink ▢	Green ▢ Pink ▢ Mauve ▢ Blue ▢ Orange ▢ Yellow Ochre ▢

Your Color Chart

Best Cosmetic & Fashion Colors to Select for Your Skin, Hair, Eyes, and Total Look

Skin Color/Undertone	Hair Colors
Medium Skin/Dark Yellow-Brown-Red	*Brown*
Crimson ▨ Deep Burgundy ▨	Green ▨ Yellow Ochre ▨
Blue Violet ▨ Deep Green ▨	Burnt Sienna ▨ Thalo Green ▨
Blue ▨ Orange ▨ Red ▨	Burnt Orange ▨ Light Crimson ▨
Wine ▨ Burnt Sienna ▨	Green ▨
Thalo Green ▨ Pink ▨	
White ☐ Gold ▨	
Dark Skin/Yellow-Brown-Red	*Brown/Dark Brown*
Russet ▨ Yellow Green ▨	Light Red ▨ Yellow ☐
Light Burnt Umber ▨	White ☐ Sand ☐ Yellow Ochre ▨
Permanent Green ▨	Light Alzarin Crimson ▨ Green ▨
Cadmium Orange ▨	Red ▨ Gold ▨ Copper ▨
Thalo Blue ▨ White ☐ Plum ▨	Fawn ▨ Deep Blue ▨
Bronze ▨ Gold ▨	Deep Blue Green ▨ Olive ▨
	Medium Pink ▨
Dark Skin/Red Blue	*Very Dark Brown*
White ☐ Cadmium Orange ▨	Cadmium Yellow ☐ Pale Yellow ☐
Permanent Green ▨ Pink ▨	Light Red ▨ Alzarin Crimson ▨
Pale Blue ▨ Red Violet ▨	Yellow Ochre ▨ Cadmium Orange ▨
Pale Green ▨	Black ▨ White ☐ Light Green ▨

Your Color Chart

Best Cosmetic & Fashion Colors to Select for Your Skin, Hair, Eyes, and Total Look

Eye Color	Best Cosmetic & Fashion Colors for Your Total Look
Brown/Dark Brown Burnt Sienna ▨ English Red ▨ Light Green ▨ Thalo Blue ▨ Crimson ☐ Pale Yellow ▨ White ☐ Cadmium Orange ▨	Crimson ▨ Orange ▨ Green ▨ White ☐
Dark Brown Orange ▨ Yellow ☐ Pale Green ☐ Orange Red ▨ Permanent Green ▨ Cadmium Yellow ☐ Light Crimson ▨ White ☐ Brown Orange ▨ Gray ▨ Pale Blue ▨ Alzarin Crimson ▨ Black ▨ Ultra Mauve ▨ Blue ▨	Green ▨ Blue ▨ Gold ▨
Dark Brown/Black Yellow ☐ White ☐ Green ▨ Alzarin Crimson ▨ Cadmium Yellow ▨ Pale & Medium Yellow Ochre ▨ Light Gray ▨	White ☐ Cadmium ☐ Green ▨

With or without make-up, daily skin care is a must. Here, these lovely ladies have enhanced their natural beauty with the appropriate base and colors that contour. Viva la difference—before and after!

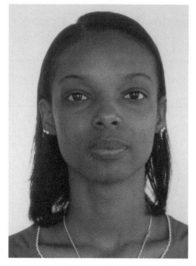 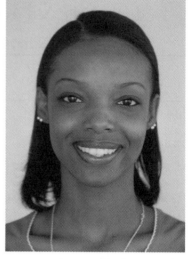

Karima Henderson   *Career Girl*

Color Plan: Rich Copper foundation with a deep shade of pressed powder, Earth-tone eye shadows in red-brown and salmon, with black eyeliner pencil and soft black mascara, Rose blusher, and red lipstick.

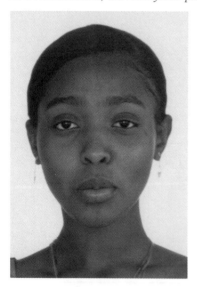 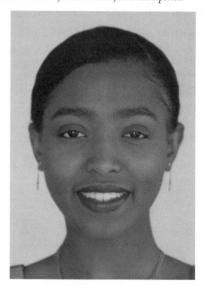

Rabiya Dumas   *College Student*

Color Plan: Deep Bronze foundation with powder, Smoky Bronze and Medium Tan eyeshadow, with black eyeliner and mascara, Rustique blusher, and Russet Red lipstick.

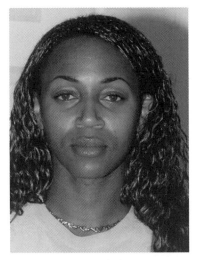

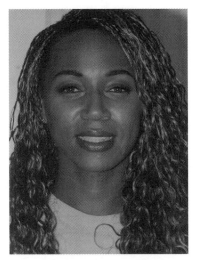

Lena Nicholson

Flight Attendant

Color Plan: Mocha-brown foundation with powder, Bold Brown and Smoky Grey eyeshadow with blue-black liner and mascara, Deep Red blusher, and Royal Red lipstick.

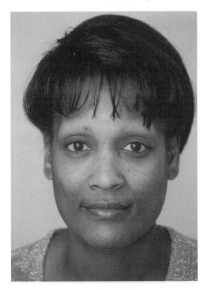

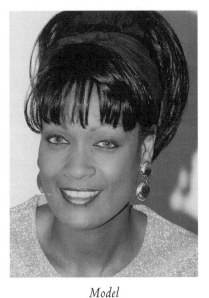

Cindy Gabbidon

Model

Color Plan: Amber foundation with powder, Soft Rose and Smoky Brown eyeshadow, with brown-black eyeliner and soft black mascara, Hot Pink blusher, and Fuchsia lipstick.

❧ Your Fabulous Lips

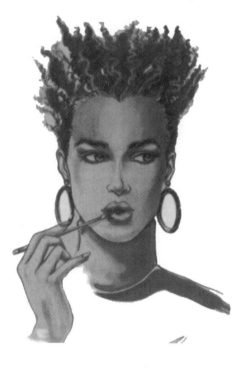

The most attractive part of an African-American women's face is her lips. No one smiles with such full lips and with such beautiful white teeth. The secure black woman who really believes that black is beautiful has no problem accepting God's gift. She flaunts her full lips when talking with a friend, communicating at work, attending religious affairs, flirting, or just being sensual.

A black woman has a natural, firm, raised lip line. The natural pout in the center and her thick upper and lower lips are attractive.

Learn how to express your lovely features by practicing before a mirror. Maximize the value and beauty of your lips. But be honest with yourself, too. If your lips have droopy, turned-down corners, teach yourself to hold the corners up. Smile more and practice looking pleasant.

Besides how you hold your lips, your mouth may have other "spoilers" needing attention—for example, missing teeth, gold teeth, yellow teeth, or poorly manufactured partial dentures. Your lips dramatically outline your mouth, therefore your teeth must not be a major negative to an otherwise beautiful face. When you have moist, dewy, luscious lips, your teeth in their whiteness and evenness only make you more inviting. Your lips, teeth, and smile make your face radiate, bringing joy to all who see you.

✤ Lip Color Options

If you are a woman who prefers just a hint of natural color (earth tones to soft beige, or pink tones), I have a suggestion: even out discolorations with concealer or your foundation base and set with powder. If your upper and lower lips are dark and even, for best results select a lip shade lighter than your lips.

You might wish to apply a lipstick product from a tube, wand, pan, or pot. There are lip glosses designed for African-American women—that is, deeply pigmented colors—that can be worn alone; they impart a moist, sheer sheen to your lips. Or you might wish to wear a clear lip gloss or lip moisturizer. This, too, would be appropriate. Don't use greasy, nonpenetrating petroleum jelly, however. It looks and feels tacky on your lips. You might want to take the time to use a lip pencil, for it is excellent in achieving a natural look. If you use a lip pencil, lightly line the lip and fill in with the pencil, covering any uneven tones, then apply a clear red, a brown lip shade, or clear tint gloss.

If you are conservative but want a pulled-together look, I suggest the medium-tone creams (clear red, russet-red, radiant red, cocoa-copper, cinnamon, café, brandied coral, raspberry, spice sienna, and so on).

Black skin usually looks best in shades of beige, yellow, yellow-brown, and blue. But consult the color chart in the photo insert before selecting a lipstick. For example, if you are of medium tone with yellow-brown skin and a sallow aura, lipsticks with a beige or deep yellow base will drain color from your skin. On the other hand, you can wear deep orange shades such as cinnamon-orange, burnt orange, radiant red, bronze-coral) and claret.

✤ Lipstick Tools

Now let's consider the lipstick tools and materials: lip liner pencil, lip brush, lip light, lip toner or foundation, and lip balancer.

1. *Lip Liner Pencil.* Liner pencils define the line of the lips and should be chosen with your skin tone in mind. For example, if you have fair to light skin) your liner should be rose-pink, light red, light plum, or light brown. Women with medium skin tones are best

using liner pencils in shades of red, light brown, brown, and plum. Those with dark skin tones look best using red, deep brown, raspberry, plum, or brown-black liners. *Never* use a black pencil to line your lips. It's unattractive and appears harsh.

When you want a new look for your lips, use a lip pencil to outline it. Lightly outline the lips and fill in the corners if your lips are full, and then edge in your selected color. The pencil should match as closely as possible the desired lip color.

Black women often have deep folds in their lips that extend to the outer edges. Lip color frequently cakes and peels to these edges, giving the appearance of bleeding color. The lip liner pencil keeps lip color from bleeding and gives a more precise lip line. When matte, oil-free pencils are used as a base for cream or frosted lipsticks, the color stays put and wears much longer.

2. *Lip Brush.* The purpose of a lipstick brush is to transfer lipstick from the tube to the surface of the lips in a smooth application. Most black women have very deep folds, or lines, in their lips. When lipstick is applied directly from the tube, the tube rides over the deep folds. The lip brush prevents this from happening, because, owing to its flexibility, the brush gets color into the crevices as well, giving a smooth, full-color application. The lipstick brush also gives you the option of lining your lips (see previous item), reducing the possibility of your lipstick bleeding once the large area is colored.

   A lipstick brush may be either man-made, of natural fibers, or a combination of both. I prefer a blend of natural and man-made fibers.

3. *Lip Light.* Lip light is a lip color adjuster, which reflects light colors away from ruddy, bluish, or very dark lips; it is worn under the lipstick.

4. *Lip Toner.* A lip toner, or foundation, is a lip adjuster that corrects slightly discolored lips, evens out lip tones, and keeps color true. Toners come in fair-to-medium and medium-to-dark shades.

5. *Lip Balancer.* A lip balancer is a deep, waxy, purplish teak natural pigment, designed to camouflage the resistant light pink discoloration often found on medium and dark lips. A lip balancer also neutralizes the acidity that causes discoloration in the center of the bottom lip, an area which is more often affected than the upper. In the process, it prevents the lipstick from changing color when placed on this area. A lip balancer is worn under the lipstick. It is excellent for subtle, medium, and deep shades of lipstick; however, the bright reds, orange-browns, and light berry shades are affected by a lip balancer.

Types of Lipstick

Lipstick types are very personal preferences, and it is up to you which you select. Lipsticks with specially formulated conditioners, moisturizers, waxes, and light mineral oil are superior to those without them, since these ingredients smooth the lips, help retain moisture, help prevent infection, and often protect sensitive skin.

Here's a special beauty note: most lipstick formulas include conditioners and emollients. For example, lip moisturizers often contain PABA (a sunscreen) along with vitamins A and E. So there are advantages over and above beauty for using a lipstick.

Now, let's review some of the major types of lipstick available today:

1. *Cream Lipsticks.* Standard cream lipsticks are deep pigment colors without shine. They wear longer and impart more coverage than the noncream sticks owing to their heavy wax base. A second cream formula is more lightweight in texture and does not feel as heavy on the lips, but it also does not wear as long because it usually has a mineral oil base.

2. *Frosted Lipsticks.* Frosted lipsticks are usually heavy pigment colors with an iridescent, pearlized, or opaque gold coverage. Black women look best in iridescent gold eye shadow, highlights, blusher highlights in gold, and most certainly lipsticks with a gold or yellow base.

3. *Silver Sparkling Frost.* Silver sparkling frost usually looks ridiculous if applied to dark or very dark skin. This is because it imparts an ashy gray look to red-brown or bluish brown skin undertones. I frown on using silver frost, the same way beauty professionals discourage blue eye shadow for white women.

4. *Long-lasting Lipsticks.* There are lipsticks formulated to last far longer than regular lipsticks. New research and development has produced long-wearing, non-smear lipstick formulas approved for women of color.

5. *Matte Lipsticks.* No-shine lipstick formulas have conditioners for a non-dry look and feel.

6. *Translucent Lipsticks.* Translucent lipsticks in tubes or wands impart just a hint of color, with sheer coverage.

7. *Lip Glosses.* Glosses have a clear, shiny, transparent base. They come in pans, pots, wands, and tubes. Some have conditioners and moisturizers, and claim healing properties. They are usually worn over lipstick to impart a sheer gloss. Lip glosses can be worn alone, as well.

8. *Nonfragrance Lipsticks.* Fragrance-free lipsticks are for sensitive and acne skin. When some women have an allergic swelling, or experience an itchy, burning sensation on their lips, this may be a reaction to their lipstick. Most women sensitive to lipstick are reacting to the lanolin, fragrance, dyes, or preservatives in the formula. If this is a problem for you, buy fragrance-free, dermatologically tested, hypoallergenic lipstick.

❦ Applying Lip Color

The lip brush is used to pick up a small amount of lip color, and then to outline the lips, filling in from the center of the mouth to the outer edges. The following is the procedure I suggest for having beautifully colored lips:

1. Apply a lip color adjuster, such as lip light.

2. Outline your lips with a sharp lip liner pencil.

3. Edge in the lipstick color along the pencil outline and coat the lips, starting with the bottom and moving to the upper lip. Apply more color in the center, moving outward to the edges. If your lips are smooth, apply color directly from the tube.

4. Add lip gloss for a moist effect or gleam.

See the illustrations that follow for specific techniques.

Full, puckered lips with lines. Your full lips usually have an attractive ridge that gives them a definite lip line. Cover your lips with foundation, preferably an oil-free formula. Blot with oil-free setting powder.

Most of us have lined, curved, crinkly lips. For best results, edge in a faint lip line with a lip brush or a lip pencil bay a shade darker (light and medium brown, red, and berry hues) for aesthetic illusions. Follow with a lip brush to produce a smooth appearance; gently stretch your lips with your index finger and draw in a smooth line. Top lip brush with gloss.

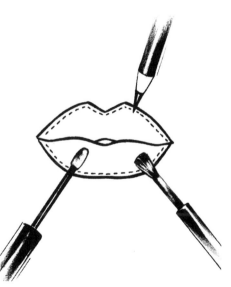

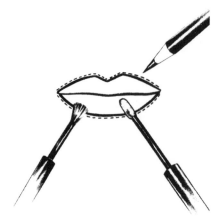

Thin lips. Cover the lips and edges with foundation. Set with oil-free powder. Redefine the lip shape you want with a lip liner pencil in a shade darker than your selected lipstick color. Fill in with lipstick and add a touch of gloss to give a moist, dewy appearance.

When one lip is larger than the other, apply foundation over the larger lip, set with oil-free powder, then edge in a line inside your natural lip line with a pencil or brush. Fill in with lipstick. Now follow the natural lip line of the smaller lip with a pencil or brush, and fill in with lipstick.

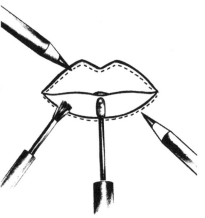

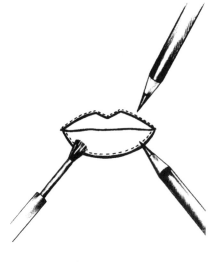

Unbalanced and droopy lips. Cover the ,even lips with foundation, and set with oil-free powder. Balance the uneven lip portion by straightening the lip line with a pencil, using a shade darker than your selected lipstick color. Blot with powder. Fill in with lipstick color.

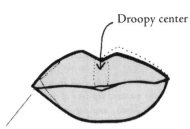

Droopy center

Droopy corners

To balance a droopy center, apply medium shade of oil-free concealer vertically through the center of the droop. Outline with pencil and lip brush, and fill in with lipstick. To cover the natural lip line at the corner, edge in with a medium dark oil-free cover stick. Blot with powder.

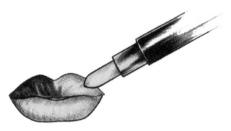

To lift a corner to create an optical illusion, use a lip pencil to extend the lower lip, taking the line upward. Continue the line just a bit above the upper lip corner. Now, extend the upper lip line to meet it. Blot with powder and fill in with lipstick color. Use a pencil, impossible.

Discolored lips. You have four options:
1. Use lip light to reflect light evenly away from uneven dark lips.
2 . Use oil-free lip toner or foundation to even out lip color.
3. Use lip balancer as a natural stain to even out acid buildup on the pink discoloration. Lip balancer will interfere with light lipstick shade,.
4. Use a medium to dark oil-free cover stick to help even out discolored lips.

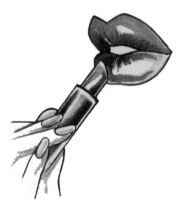

Dry, crinkly, lined lips. Condition lips with gloss or lip moisturizer which contains mineral oil, cocoa butter, phenol, alum, camphor, and beeswax.

👉 Five-Minute Face

The following order of make-up application should be followed:
1. *Moisturize*
2. *Add foundation*
3. *Set foundation with powder*
4. *Do eyes: one color eyelid and eye color application*
5. *Apply mascara*
6. *Brush eyebrows*
7. *Add lipstick color*

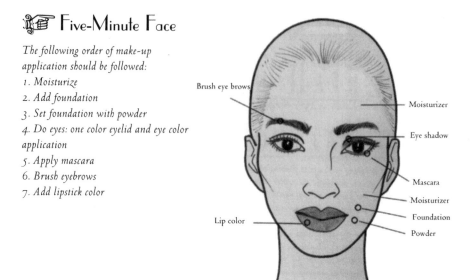

👉 Ten-Minute Face

Use the following order to apply make-up:
1. *Moisturize*
2. *Add foundation*
3. *Apply powder to set foundation*
4. *Do eyes: apply eye concealer, highlight brow bone with color, contour center of eyelid with color; apply fashion eye color to area closest to eyelash; apply eye liner, mascara; brush eyebrow and apply brow pencil*
5. *Apply blusher*
6. *Apply lip color*

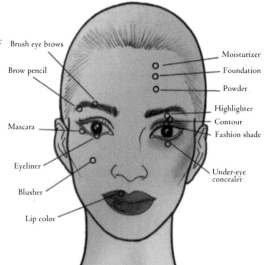

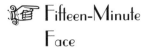

Fifteen-Minute Face

Use the following order to apply make-up:

1. *Moisturize*
2. *Apply under-eye concealer*
3. *Apply foundation*
4. *Apply powder to set foundation*
5. *Do eyes: for rainbow eyes, apply fashion shade to under corner of eye, highlight the center point of eyelid, contour the outer corner of eyelid; apply eyeliner to top and bottom lid; use brow brush, brow pencil, mascara*
6. *Do cheeks: contour the cheek area underneath the cheekbone and then apply blusher on top of cheekbone, blending down to contour*
7. *Do lips: use lip pencil to line lips, add lip color with lip brush, and add a touch of lip gloss*

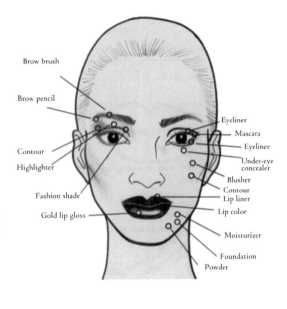

Chapter 7

Your Hair, Hands, and Nails

While a student at the nation's largest beauty education system, the Wilfred Beauty Academy in New York, I had the opportunity to learn and practice my skills on every type of hair in the world. My first position as a hair stylist was in Macy's department store in New York City. The majority of women whose hair I styled were white, from all parts of the world and with all types of hair textures. This was a learning opportunity, but I wanted experience with black hair.

A friend, Delores, and I decided that the only way we were going to get hands-on experience with African-American hair was to work in an African-American environment. So I went straight to Harlem. I was hired to work at a prestigious and elegant salon, the Rose Morgan House of Beauty.

Never before or since have I seen a beauty salon so elegantly appointed. I learned that the right hairstyle makes a woman feel more confident and secure about her total appearance. Her hair and her make-up communicate attractive and positive images to those around her. Women have told me that when they know they are well made up and their hair is just right, they feel they are on top of the world. They know they feel and look great.

❦ Black Hair is Manageable

Don't worry, your hair can readily be managed by you or your hair-stylists Black women's hairstyles and hair management have come full circle. This $4 billion beauty industry—predominantly composed of black companies—has researched and developed all types of formulas for styling and maintenance. My past work at the Rose Morgan House of Beauty and the years of experience that have followed, have taught me the following:

1. Black women retain their hair longer as they mature than any other group of people.

2. A black woman can style her hair in more ways than any other woman, including braiding, plaiting, and corn rolls.

3. Black hair has natural, built-in body owing to its curly wave pattern.

4. African-American hair comes in some thirty or more textures, based on tribal origin, from Nubian and Mandingo to African Australian.

5. Natural black hair color comes in some thirty or more gradations, from the ash blond of Samoa to the flaxen blond of New Orleans.

❦ The Right Hairstyle

Today's salon hairstylists are a refreshing new breed of creative, skillful, talented people who can make appropriate suggestions concerning your hair care, as well as cut, curl, and style your hair—all based on your facial shape.

If you consider working with your hair, keep your face in mind. Too much hair moving forward toward the center of your head, with bangs falling into your eyes will show age on your face more than any other hairstyle; hair moving away from the center of your forehead takes years off your face.

For some reason, many black women wear hairstyles that move their hair forward toward the center of the forehead, making their face appear much older and more mature than it is. Instead, reverse this apparent movement. For example, if you have a low forehead and a short neck, you can give the illusion of adding more height by styling your hair high, with medium curls on your head, and by keeping your hair away from your neck, styling it close to the sides of your head. On the other hand, when a woman's hair is long, all anyone sees is her head and shoulders; they don't see her neck. If your neck is long and you have a high forehead, style your hair to fall into soft curls, some to the side and some across the forehead in a sculptured fashion.

To help you with styling problems I have put together a collection of hairstyles that address problems with the neck, forehead, nose, jaw, and chin (see pages 126-132). These styles vary from straight or curly to corn rows and Afros. They are to excite your imagination while providing the necessary clues you can employ to camouflage a problem.

In these styles you will not find the exaggerated, short and wavy marcelled look, the fashionable ornaments and ribbons or gold jewelry adornments, or the pancake and flattop styles. Such styles are neither for you nor for the life you lead. In all cases, remember that *symmetry* and *balance* are the operative words.

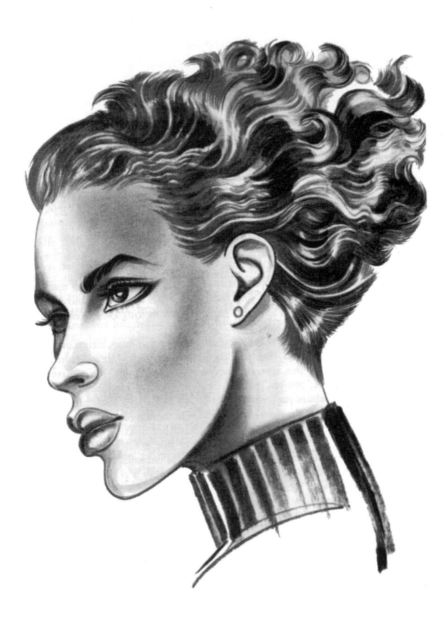

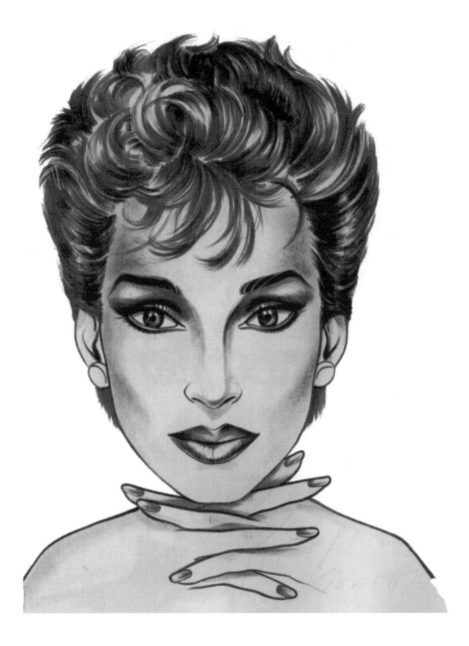

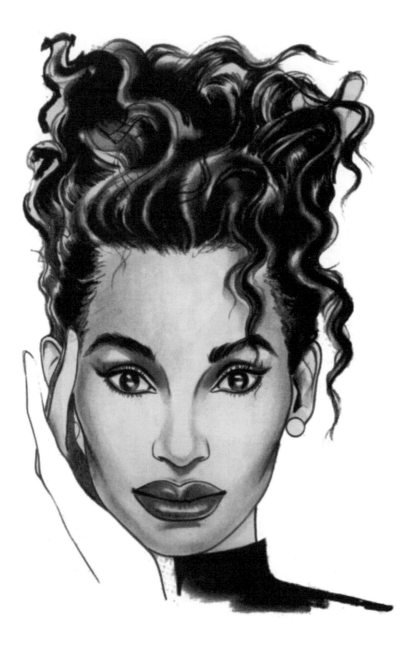

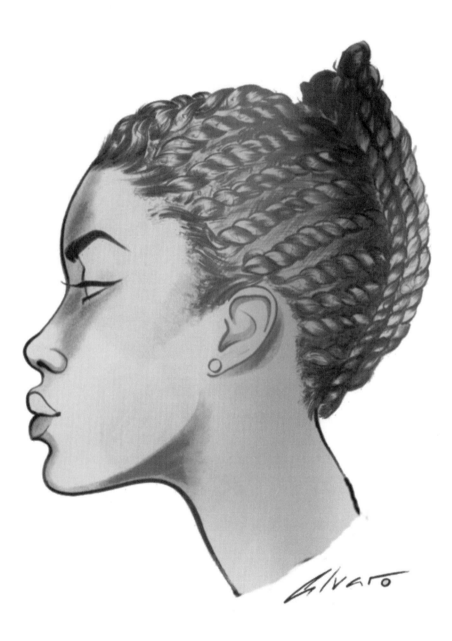

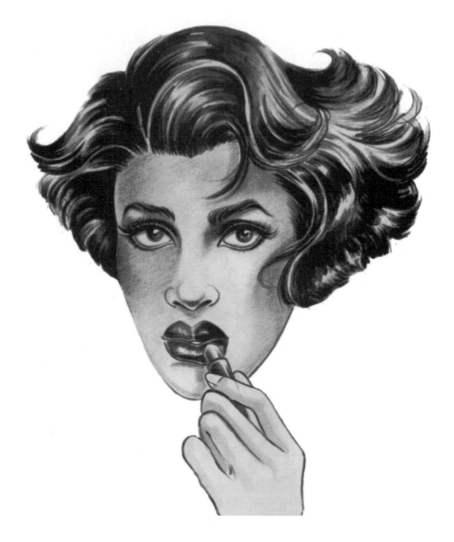

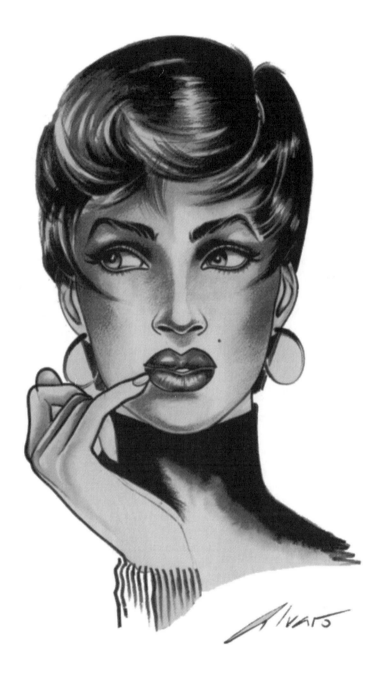

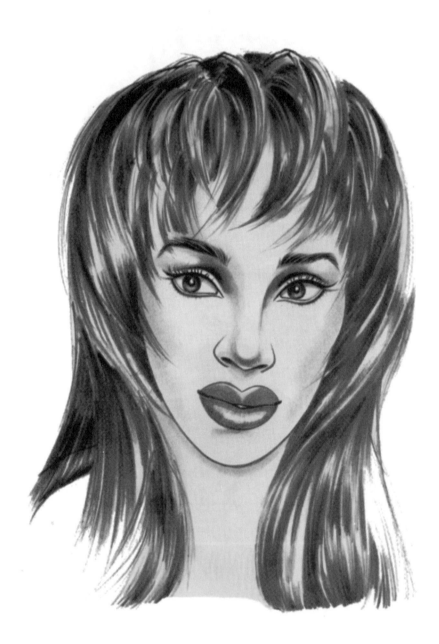

❧ Hair Shaping

The right haircut and shape is the key to an ideal hairstyle. Black women must go regularly to a professional beauty salon for shaping and cutting. Some women prefer a barber shop, but I recommend a women's salon. The lines and symmetry for women's hairstyles are entirely different from men's.

In cutting and shaping your hair, a professional should take your features and facial shape into consideration. Extreme hairstyles are not for you.

❧ Hair Color

When I was beauty editor at *Ebony* magazine, the editors of *Chain and Drug Store* magazine, a trade publication, asked me, "What were the newest trends in hair grooming products for the black woman of the '90s?" The answer was obvious: the African-American woman wanted more color in her life. Black women wanted to enhance and highlight their otherwise very dark hair. Well, what was perceived as a trend then is now an avalanche. I could not be happier. Today's black woman of the millennium is throwing off the shackles of dowdy conservatism and using color.

No longer is it just black companies that are preparing hair products for blacks. Clairol's innovative Instant Water conditioning beauty shampoo-in formula and Dark and Lovely's conditioning formulas, and Revlon's Color Style Tints are excellent examples of what is happening in the retail market. My favorite new hair colorings are the fabulous berry shades that range from strawberry to plum. And the rich bronzes and browns with apricot-cinnamon and chestnut highlights are fabulous, and some blondes do have more fun, too. Variety is definitely here!

Like your skin undertone, your hair has a tone that ranges from yellow-gold or yellow-red to red, dark red, or red-brown, and to brown--black. Your skin tone, eye color, and natural hair color are your best guides in choosing a correct hair color. Remember: you have my color chart in the photo insert to help you. You also have help available from your beauty-salon hair colorist and the manufacturer's information in the insert and on the back of the hair coloring package.

The best guide to choosing a hair color, however, is a hair strand test, which you can do yourself. Test a strand or section of hair to see how the new color will relate to your eyes and skin. Also determine how the change makes you feel—before going all the way. Take a strand from underneath your outer layer of hair so it won't show if you decide not to proceed. The strand test can be done under the supervision of your hair colorist or at home with an over-the-counter product.

Whichever coloring process you choose—home or salon—there are three basic types of hair color:

🐾 *Temporary color.* These are shampoo-in formulas that are nonalkaline and work gently with the natural chemistry of your hair. Temporary colors are noncoating and will not penetrate the hair shaft. Temporary colors wash out, and usually do not contain ammonia, peroxide, or other harmful ingredients.

🐾 *Semipermanent color.* These are designed to harden and coat the outer cuticle shaft of the hair. Semipermanent colors start to rinse off after four or six washings. Some semipermanent color products contain peroxide.

🐾 *Permanent color.* These change the character pigment balance and natural hair color. Permanent hair coloring is best applied in a salon by a professional hair colorist, particularly if you are insecure about your first color change. Permanent hair color products last longer than any other hair change process. Special care for treated hair is advised.

🐾 *Color crayons.* "Tween-Time Hair" and "Cover Gray" are excellent touch-up tools, made of tea, stearate, paraffin, and beeswax. Hair coloring crayons are designed to conceal the roots of your natural hair growth between temporary, semipermanent, and permanent hair colorings. You moisten the crayon and apply it to the hair shaft.

There are other natural and synthetic ways to change your hair color, including special formulas to cover gray hair, color tints, color sprays, mousses, natural henna, and comb-in hair coloring.

❧ Your Hands Are Lovely

Lovely hands can be the ultimate statement in your total grooming regimen. But making that statement requires proper care.

Your hands are constantly exposed to stresses: weather, pollutants, detergents and other irritating chemicals, and dirt. They get cut, bruised and scraped. When you clean your hands, you usually wash them in soap and water, removing the limited moisture and oils the body has provided to protect them. Your hands do not have as many oil producing glands or as much fatty tissue per square inch as does your face. There are no oil glands on the palms of your hands (sweat glands, yes). Thus, washing with drying soaps is more stressful for your hands than you probably realize.

Often, the results of poor hand care can be seen in the ashen-colored skin between the thumb and index finger, and on the knuckles and cuticles on black women. Regardless of your skin tone, dry-looking skin is unattractive. It shows up more on dark skin, and therefore black skin requires a more intensive hand-care regimen. As you would suppose, the seasons of the year affect your hands differently, and the worst season is winter.

Winter hand care usually means applying an extra-dry hand-cream formula. I do not recommend petroleum jelly, since it gives the hands a greasy, tacky look and feel. It also attracts dirt, particles to the hands and under the nails. There are excellent over-the-counter hand-care products to use, but you must use them faithfully.

Proper care of the hands also requires periodic, regular pampering, which includes a regular manicure. Learn from your manicurist and care for your hands personally between visits.

❧ Your Nails and Their Care

Let's look at some important terms before discussing nail health and care. The nail mantle is a protective plate located at the end of the finger. It is made up of the following:

1. The nail bed upon which the nail surface rests.

2. The cuticle, a thin outer layer of the nail skin epidermis.

3. The matrix, or formative intercellular tissue of the nail; blood cells nourish the matrix.

4. The lunula, or whitish half-moon shape at the base of the fingernail.

The important, often-abused cuticles serve to protect the nail and keep environmental impurities and germs away from the healthy growing nail.

Nail-Care Products and Processes

There are several terms that a manicurist uses in caring for your nails.

🕱 *Nail bleach*—a salon manicuring cosmetic used to remove stains from under the edges of the fingernail tips.

🕱 *Nail white*—a nail cosmetic used to whiten the free edge of the nail.

🕱 *Nail white pencil*—a pencil containing a hard white chalk, used to whiten the free edge underneath the fingernail tips.

🕱 *Nail enamel or polish*—a fingernail polish in the form of a liquid, which forms a colored or transparent coating on glued-on fingernails.

🕱 *Nail lacquer*—a thick liquid that forms a high glossy film on your nails.

🕱 *Nail transplants*—process by which a manicurist cements a broken fingernail to a natural nail.

🕱 *Nail extensions*—process by which a manicurist applies a premixed material at the juncture of the natural fingernail tip and the silver-foil nail form, forming and sculpting an artificially extended nail.

🕱 *Nail wrappings*—process by which the manicurist covers the nail's outer tissue, sealing it with a protective nail enamel or glaze, for a smoother, harder, and more durable nail prepared to receive enamel.

Artificial Nails

Artificial nails are out of fashion. Any health care provider experienced with hand and nail care will agree that artificial nails cause all kinds of problems for nails. Fungus infections and bacterial growth is a major concern.

Nail Health

A healthy nail grows 1/32 of an inch each week. Nails grow rapidly until you are 30, and then as you mature their growth rate decreases to one half the youthful rate. Of course, a good diet, regular exercise, and adequate water consumption will enhance the health of your nails.

Slower than normal nail growth can result in excessive thickening of the nails. Breaking, splitting, and peeling can be hereditary or can result from a dietary deficiency or nutritional imbalance. If any of these conditions worsen, consult your physician or dermatologist before your next manicure.

As strange as it may seem—except to those black women who have had first-hand experience—physicians with limited, if any, prior experience with black patients sometimes see a dark-skinned black woman with heavily pigmented nails (and dark-pigmented gums or lined pigmented eyes) or naturally, dark cuticles and indicate that there is a disease—or worse. I am so annoyed with such lazy doctors; I have to assume that they don't care to know more, for the medical data are available, telling them and the world that these are distinct racial features of many healthy African-Americans.

Your eyes, mouth, hands, and nails are mirrors of your health, and knowledgeable doctors are able to discern health vs. disease. Many normal conditions in blacks are abnormal in whites; in many instances, there is no carryover. Your physician or dermatologist should know this. Make sure the professionals who treat you are skilled, experienced, and knowledgeable about black skin and its conditions.

Also, if at any time you notice that your hands show a reddish-yellowing, with a reddish purple aura against a white background, immediately consult your doctor.

Likewise, if you have infected, sensitive crusty dark cuticles, swollen and sensitive skin at the sides of the nails and fingertips, skin discolorations, or rashes and fine bumps, you should be concerned and seek medical advice.

❦ Home Care of Your Nails

The use of chemicals, internal and topical medications, drastic diet changes, and nail color, polish removers, artificial nails, and nail base coats can often cause nail discoloration, nail breakage, dryness, and general poor nail health. If possible, wear gloves when working in the garden, washing dishes, and so on. Buff your nails on occasion, giving them a relief from the nail base and polish. Be careful with your eating habits and don't go on crash diets. Watch your medication; don't be pill happy, as so many of us are. Good nutrition and proper vitamin supplements will help keep your nails healthy while doing wonders for your entire system.

Regularly consult a professional manicurist. Ask your manicurist to teach you how to care for your hands and nails in between visits. In addition, to help you care for your nails, I have prepared a basic at-home program. You will need a bowl of warm, sudsy water; a bowl of clear water; and towels.

Hand and Nail Wardrobe

Assemble the following items:

1. Polish remover—a fragrance-free, oil-based formula without acetone.

2. Nail file—wood or metal for shaping and cleaning.

3. Cream or liquid cuticle remover—aids in the removal of dead skin around cuticles.

4. Cuticle stick—to gently push back the cuticles.

5. Base coat—holds the color on the nail.

6. Top coat—seals the color in and protects the surface.

7. Nail polish—coloring as follows: cream for all occasions; high lacquer gloss for glamorous occasions, and frost for every occasion.

8. Cotton balls—large balls for nail cleaning and polish removal.

You should also have a hand cream designed for manicure use and cuticle cream for nightly cuticle protection.

❧ How to Select Nail Color

Your nail color should match your lipstick—that is, blue nails do not go with red lipstick. Pick up your fashion cues from your garments. Also, consult the color chart in the photo insert.

Procedure

There are two possible methods. The first is to remove any old polish and apply nail cream, then buff your nails. The second method is to remove the polish, apply a clear base coat, and a tinted polish, then add a top coat.

Chapter 8

Skin Care and Grooming for Men

It is women who more often than not choose the clothes that men wear, and men more often "dress up" to please women than other men. Women are also more inclined to buy and read a book like this. Consequently, I include this chapter for men with the hope that you will share it with the men in your life.

More and more, though, men are realizing that proper grooming is not a luxury or simply a personal desire. It is a necessity. Men of color are finding themselves performing professional roles where appearance is a critical element of success. They find themselves in positions that call for a suit and tie, such as business meetings, and to be photographed for print media and for television, as well as for social occasions. Whatever the reason, this is a basic skin-care and grooming guide for men who want to look their best and for those who want the most sensible solutions for dealing with their particular needs and problems.

Men of color—particularly men of African descent—like women, have special problems and challenges where skin care and grooming are concerned. The most frequent concerns are skin problems from razor bumps or ingrown hairs and hair care in general.

❧ Razor Bumps and Other Skin Problems

Razor bumps happen when very curly and wiry facial hair, cut at the wrong angle, curves over and into the skin. These bumps are itchy, painful, and can become infected. Once they become infected they can result in keloids—scar tissue—and leave marks and pits in the skin. These razor bumps pose chronic problems for many men and lead many of them to decide to wear beards, opting not to shave at all. Beards can look great, but you should wear one because you want to and not because you feel you have to. Alternatively, there are some shaving techniques whereby you can have a clean-shaven look without the discomfort of razor bumps.

There are preconditioners—gels, foams, liquids, and steam—that soften the beard and set it up for cutting. There are razors with special heads and blades that cut hairs at such an angle that they are less likely to curl over and into the skin. If you have a difficult beard and are susceptible to razor bumps, a single- or twin-blade razor, or a straight-edge razor in the hands of your barber, is best. Many black men, though, find that electric razors nick, cause bumps, and irritate sensitive skin. Curly hair should be shaved in one direction. The electric razor does not cut hair in one direction, and this is how it causes problems.

Some men try depilatories in their attempt to avoid shaving problems. If this is your choice, use those designed for sensitive black skin and capable of removing hair without irritation and burning, like Easy Shave Medicated Shave Cream—which is a preconditioner and moisturizer which concentrates on healing razor bumps—Magic Shave Depilatory from the Carson Products Company, Black Opal's Shaving System, the Edgar Morris Corrective Shaving Kit, and the E.T. Browne Drug Company's facial depilatory that includes cocoa butter. Some of the products good for preconditioning your skin for shaving are razor burn products—antibiotic cream, mild hydrocortisone, and Neosporin combined with Cortaid—Clinique's Post Shave Healer, Eclipse Razor Relief Balm, Aramis Lab Series Razor Burn Relief, and the Black Opal Shaving System is highly recommended.

❧ Beards

If you are going to wear a beard, it should be regularly cleaned, conditioned, brushed or combed, and designed for your facial bone structure. Actually, a beard helps keep the skin looking younger because the hairs protect the skin from sun damage. The hairs will also keep the skin from folding, therefore the skin will have fewer wrinkles. Acne problems are also less of a problem for men with beards. Consult a good barber to determine the appropriate shape of the beard for your bone structure.

❧ A Skin-Care Regimen

Attending to your face requires but minutes a day. Refer to Chapters 1 through 3 to learn how to establish a skin-care regimen that suits your skin type. Cleanse, tone, and moisturize are the key steps to healthy and great-looking skin for men, too.

I strongly recommend that men treat themselves to facials, periodically. Not only are they good for keeping the skin moisturized and healthy, but they help you to relieve tension. Getting a facial can offer you a peaceful time when you can relax those facial muscles. Adequate sleep, plenty of water, annual medical check-ups, and sound daily nutritional habits are important as well.

❧ Hair Grooming

There has never been a time when the African-American male has had more hairstyle options. Yet this very fact has added an issue every professional adult male must address if he wishes to move effectively and smoothly from the boardroom or TV station into the playing field or other social setting.

Just as the style and color of your clothes can admit you to or keep you out of certain places, so can your hairstyle. Certain hairstyles are acceptable in the entertainment world but not in the executive boardrooms of Wall Street and Park Avenue. Styles that make you "hip" in social situations may be counterproductive in terms of your business career. The style that is in fashion may also be inappropriate for your face.

When it comes to choosing a hairstyle, look for one that will fit the most critical aspects of your life. For example, if you choose the latest fad styles, you are making a clear nonconservative, nonbusiness statement, and you should expect to be viewed, if not treated, accordingly.

The best general hairstyle is still the classic look, a reasonably cropped style which tapers gently downward to the sides and nape of the neck, with a clean neckline. This style can be just as natural and appropriate by wearing your hair somewhat fuller overall or by employing gentle, full waves with the hair somewhat longer at the nape of the neck. Another variation is to have the temples fuller and nape fuller. This style is great if you have large ears or if they stand away from the head. Having a fuller top elongates the face.

If you are patterned bald or balding, wear your hair closely cropped. This reduces the look of baldness. To retard the balding process, Cleanse your hair at least once a week with a shampoo formulated for your type of hair. Massage your hair daily with your fingertips to stimulate the blood flow. This will help feed the hair follicles.

When shampooing your hair, always apply a conditioner after shampooing and wash it out after about five minutes. Leaving it in longer will not hurt, but it will not do any more good. Before your hair is styled, it should always be shampooed. If you have coarse hair, you may want a mild relaxer applied before your shampoo and styling. But if you use a relaxer, be sure to use an acid-neutralized shampoo.

Do not forget that hair texture for black males comes in as many varieties as black skin color, and it will therefore need different treatments. If you want a modern rather than a classic look, have your hair processed with a curly perm, giving it a sheen and high manageability. If you use chemicals on your hair, it becomes more susceptible to damage; therefore, such hair must be properly conditioned and periodically rested from chemicals to maintain its health.

But whatever your hair type or perceived problem, there is a product to assist you, from relaxers to curlers, from toupees to weaves, from transplants to glue-ons or braids—all giving you the look of a natural, full head of hair. Think first about the look you want and its consequences to both your total image and your lifestyle before choosing it.

Conclusion

I have found that everyone seems to have something to say about the African-American woman, but no one seems to be listening to her. Cosmetic companies and general market beauty and fashion magazines tend to take too narrow a view of both black beauty culture and black style, often pursuing its own policies and point of view, without acting as a true reflection of our complex African-American generation. Our generation is different from previous ones. The industry is finally recognizing the African-American woman's 21st century beauty needs and realizing that she doesn't just have one beauty image appearance; she has many beauty looks.

African-American women have, within their souls, potentialities that can be discovered and nurtured to help them become more attractive, more interesting, and more appealing persons. *The African-American Woman's Guide to Successful Make-up and Skin Care* was written and designed specifically to help you make the most of these potentialities so that you can achieve success and happiness, both in your work and in your personal life.

I have had the opportunity to travel all over this world to observe and touch beautiful women of African heritage. I've enjoyed sharing with you my experience and you have taught me to respect and appreciate your ageless beauty.

This basic beauty guide expresses the needs and wants of the 21st century African-American woman, who is dynamic and assured with strong family values, by providing perspectives on her beauty and her total beauty image in the workplace.

You, the readers, are the intended audience of *The African-American Woman's Guide to Successful Make-up and Skin Care*—women with buying power and influence, who work for their style of living and that of their families.

I look forward to meeting you soon.

Alfred Fornay

Appendix 1

Your Personal Skin Care Chart

Season

❏ Fall ❏ Winter ❏ Spring ❏ Summer

Type of Skin

❏ Oily ❏ Dry ❏ Combination ❏ Sensitive

Day Care

Cleanse _____

Tone _____

Moisturize _____

Eye treatment _____

Night Care

Special night treatment _____

Weekly Treatment

Mask _____

Scrub _____

Firming cream _____

Special skin-bleaching cream _____

Your Personal Color Chart

Season

❑ Fall   ❑ Winter   ❑ Spring   ❑ Summer

Type of Skin

❑ Oily   ❑ Dry   ❑ Combination   ❑ Sensitive

Foundation

Liquid color

Cream color   _____

Concealer

Cover stick

Concealer   _____

Eye colors: _____

Eyeliner: _____

Mascara colors: _____

Eyebrow colors: _____

Blusher: _____

Contour shade: _____

Cheek highlighter: _____

Day lip colors: _____

Night lip colors: _____

Lip color adjuster: _____

Lip moisturizer: _____

Sheer lip tint: _____

Lip gloss: _____

Index

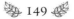

ORDER FORM

Fax Orders: 602-283-0991
Telephone Orders: 602-460-1660
Online Orders: E-mail: Amberbk@aol.com
Postal Orders: Send Checks and Money Orders to:
                Amber Books Publishing
                1334 East Chandler Blvd., Suite 5-D67
                Phoenix, AZ 85048

Please send _____ copy/ies of "The African-American Woman's Guide to Successful Make-up and Skin Care by Alfred Fornay.

Please send _____ copy/ies of "How to Play the Sports Recruiting Game and Get an Athletic Scholarship: The Handbook and Guide to Success for the African-American High School Student-Athlete" by Rodney J. McKissic.

Please send _____ copy/ies of "Is Modeling for You? The Handbook and Guide for the Young Aspiring Black Model" by Yvonne Rose and Tony Rose.

Name:_____

Company Name:_____

Address:_____

City:_____State:_____Zip:_____

Telephone: (_____) _____

        Successful Make-up $14.95
        Sports Recruiting: $12.95
        Modeling: $14.95

❏ Check   ❏ Money Order   ❏ Cashiers Check
Payable to Amber Books, 1334 E. Chandler Blvd., Suite 5-D67, Phoenix, AZ 85048

Shipping: $5.00 per book. Allow 7 days for delivery.
Sales Tax: Add 7.05% to books shipped to Arizona addresses.
Total enclosed: $_____

For Bulk Rates Call: 602-460-1660

ORDER NOW

ORDER FORM

Fax Orders: 602-283-0991
Telephone Orders: 602-460-1660
Online Orders: E-mail: Amberbk@aol.com
Postal Orders: Send Checks and Money Orders to:
                Amber Books Publishing
                1334 East Chandler Blvd., Suite 5-D67
                Phoenix, AZ 85048

Please send _____ copy/ies of "The African-American Woman's Guide to Successful Make-up and Skin Care by Alfred Fornay.

Please send _____ copy/ies of "How to Play the Sports Recruiting Game and Get an Athletic Scholarship: The Handbook and Guide to Success for the African-American High School Student-Athlete" by Rodney J. McKissic.

Please send _____ copy/ies of "Is Modeling for You? The Handbook and Guide for the Young Aspiring Black Model" by Yvonne Rose and Tony Rose.

Name:_____

Company Name:_____

Address:_____

City:_____State:_____Zip:_____

Telephone: (_____) _____

Successful Make-up	$14.95
Sports Recruiting:	$12.95
Modeling:	$14.95

❏ Check ❏ Money Order ❏ Cashiers Check
Payable to Amber Books, 1334 E. Chandler Blvd., Suite 5-D67, Phoenix, AZ 85048

Shipping: $5.00 per book. Allow 7 days for delivery.
Sales Tax: Add 7.05% to books shipped to Arizona addresses.
Total enclosed: $_____

For Bulk Rates Call: 602-460-1660

ORDER NOW

ORDER FORM

Fax Orders: 602-283-0991
Telephone Orders: 602-460-1660
Online Orders: E-mail: Amberbk@aol.com
Postal Orders: Send Checks and Money Orders to:
               Amber Books Publishing
               1334 East Chandler Blvd., Suite 5-D67
               Phoenix, AZ 85048

Please send _____ copy/ies of "The African-American Woman's Guide to Successful Make-up and Skin Care by Alfred Fornay.

Please send _____ copy/ies of "How to Play the Sports Recruiting Game and Get an Athletic Scholarship: The Handbook and Guide to Success for the African-American High School Student-Athlete" by Rodney J. McKissic.

Please send _____ copy/ies of "Is Modeling for You? The Handbook and Guide for the Young Aspiring Black Model" by Yvonne Rose and Tony Rose.

Name:_____

Company Name:_____

Address:_____

City:_____State:_____Zip:_____

Telephone: (_____) _____

       Successful Make-up $14.95
       Sports Recruiting: $12.95
       Modeling: $14.95

❑ Check   ❑ Money Order   ❑ Cashiers Check
Payable to Amber Books, 1334 E. Chandler Blvd., Suite 5-D67, Phoenix, AZ 85048

Shipping: $5.00 per book. Allow 7 days for delivery.
Sales Tax: Add 7.05% to books shipped to Arizona addresses.
Total enclosed: $_____

For Bulk Rates Call: 602-460-1660

ORDER NOW

A SPECIAL OFFER!

❦ FORNAY

the newsletter of beauty • culture • cosmetics
• hair • fragrance • personal appearance

I would like to give you a personal invitation to join a select circle of subscribers in getting the latest news about cosmetic foundation and color, skin care products and regimens, hair color, hair treatment and management, the latest hairstyles, professional profiles of key make-up artists, hairstylists, nail and handcare personnel, and the fragrance echelon.

This is my newsletter. As the Publisher and Editor-in-Chief, I assure you the same quality in production and articles that you have received from me in the past.

The newsletter will be published six times a year at the subscription price of $12.00. The first issue will be published Spring/April 1999. If you subscribe in advance, the price is $10.00. Subscribe today!

Name:_____

Address:_____Apt.#:_____

City:_____State:_____Zip:_____

(Optional) Telephone #: (____)_____

(Optional) Occupation:_____

What would you like to see in upcoming newsletters?_____

_____

Send to: FORNAY
                Post Office Box 1321
                Grand Central Station, New York 10163-1321

Notes

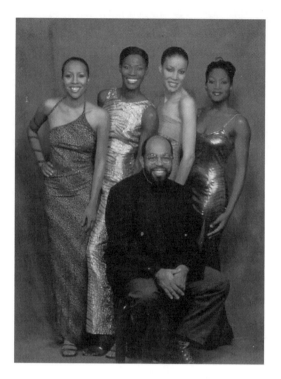

Mr. Fornay is one of the leading recognized authorities on fashion, beauty, and grooming. A graduate of the State University of New York's Fashion Institute of Technology and The University of New York, with degrees in merchandising and marketing, Mr. Fornay has influenced the marketing and sales strategies of major cosmetics firms, such as Fashion Fair, Clairol, and Revlon. As exemplified by cover models: Greer, Ericka, Judith, and Cecily, Alfred Fornay is the "New Guru" of make-up and skin care for a new generation of black women the world over.